W9-CCK-579

Selective COX-2 Inhibitors

Pharmacology, Clinical Effects and Therapeutic Potential

The publishers are grateful to
Dr Michelle Browner,
Roche Bioscience, Palo Alto, California,
for the schematic diagram of the
human COX-2 dimer shown on the cover

Selective COX-2 Inhibitors

Pharmacology, Clinical Effects and Therapeutic Potential

Edited by

SIR JOHN VANE and DR JACK BOTTING

*The William Harvey Research Institute, Saint Bartholomew's
and the Royal London School of Medicine and Dentistry,
Charterhouse Square, London, United Kingdom*

*Proceedings of a conference held
on March 20–21, 1997
in Cannes, France*

The conference organisers wish to thank

**Boehringer
Ingelheim**

for an educational grant to support this conference

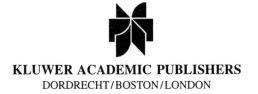

KLUWER ACADEMIC PUBLISHERS
DORDRECHT / BOSTON / LONDON

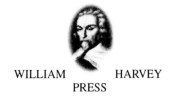

WILLIAM   HARVEY
PRESS

Distributors

for the United States and Canada: Kluwer Academic Publishers, PO Box 358, Accord Station, Hingham, MA 02018–0358, USA
for all other countries: Kluwer Academic Publishers Group, Distribution Center, PO Box 322, 3300 AH Dordrecht, The Netherlands

A catalogue record for this book is available from the Library of Congress.

ISBN 0–7923–8729–5

Copyright

© 1998 by Kluwer Academic Publishers and William Harvey Press

All rights reserved. No part of this publication may be reproduced, stored in a retrieval system, or transmitted in any form or by any means, electronic, mechanical, photocopying, recording or otherwise, without prior permission from the publishers, Kluwer Academic Publishers BV, PO Box 17, 3300 AA Dordrecht, The Netherlands.

Published in the United Kingdom by Kluwer Academic Publishers, PO Box 55, Lancaster, UK, and William Harvey Press, Charterhouse Square, London, UK.

Printed in Great Britain.

Contents

List of Contributors

Nicolas G. Bazan
Neuroscience Center of Excellence, Louisiana State University, Medical Center, School of Medicine, 2020 Gravier Street, New Orleans, LA 70112, USA.
Co-authors: Victor Marcheselli, Pranab Mukherjee, Walter Lukiw, William Gordon and Daoling Zhang

Michelle F. Browner
Molecular Structure Department, Roche Bioscience, 3401 Hillview Avenue, Palo Alto, CA 94303, USA.

Raymond N. DuBois
Department of Medicine, Vanderbilt University Medical Center, Nashville, TN 37232–2279, USA.
Co-authors: Hongmiao Sheng, Jinyi Shao, Christopher Williams and Daniel Beauchamp

Helmut Fenner
Swiss Federal Institute of Technology, Zürich, Switzerland.

Anthony Ford-Hutchinson
Merck Frosst Centre for Therapeutic Research, 16711 Trans Canada Highway, Kirkland, Quebec H9H 3L1, Canada.

Jürgen C. Frölich
Institute of Clinical Pharmacology, Hannover Medical School, 30623 Hannover, Germany.
Co-author: Dirk O. Stichtenoth

Daniel E. Furst
Arthritis Clinical Research Unit, Virginia Mason Research Center, 1000 Seneca Street, Seattle, WA 98101, USA.

Ryszard J. Gryglewski
Department of Pharmacology, Jagiellonian University Medical College, Grzegórzecka 16, 31–531 Cracow, Poland.

Christopher J. Hawkey
Division of Gastroenterology, University Hospital, Nottingham NG7 2UH, UK.

Philip Needleman
G. D. Searle Research and Development, 700 Chesterfield Village Parkway, St Louis, MO 63198, USA.
Co-authors: Peter Isakson, Ben Zweifel, Jaime Masferrer, Carol Koboldt, Karen Seibert, Richard Hubbard and Steven Geis

Michel Pairet
Department of Biological Research, Boehringer Ingelheim Research & Development, Birkendorfer Str. 65, 88397 Biberach a/d Riss, Germany.
Co-authors: Joanne van Ryn, Annerose Mauz, Hans Schierok, Willi Diederen, Dietrich Türck and Günther Engelhardt

Carlo Patrono
Center for Experimental Therapeutics, University of Pennsylvania, 905 Stellar-Chance Laboratories, 422 Curie Boulevard, Philadelphia, PA 19104–61100, USA.
Co-authors: Francesco Cipollone, Giulia Renda and Paola Patrignani

Daniel L. Simmons
Department of Chemistry and Biochemistry, E280 BNSN, Brigham Young University, Provo, UT 84602, USA.
Co-authors: Matthew Madsen and Philip Robertson

John R. Vane
The William Harvey Research Institute, St Bartholomew's and the Royal London School of Medicine and Dentistry, Queen Mary and Westfield College, Charterhouse Square, London EC1M 6BQ, UK.
Co-author: Regina Botting

Preface

The mainstay of therapy for rheumatoid disease is the non-steroid antiinflammatory drugs (NSAIDs), despite their inherent gastrointestinal toxicity and ability to cause renal damage in susceptible patients. The theory that the beneficial and toxic effects of NSAIDs stem from a reduction in prostanoid production through inhibition of cyclooxygenase implied that particular toxicities were inevitable with NSAIDs and would always be correlated with efficacy. However, over the years, it became apparent that at therapeutic doses, some NSAIDs had greater toxic side-effects than others, a fact not explained by the general theory. A significant clarification arose from the discovery that there are two distinct isoforms of COX, a constitutive enzyme (COX-1) responsible for the production of prostanoids necessary for platelet aggregation and protection of the gastric mucosa and kidney; and an inducible enzyme (COX-2) that is newly synthesized at sites of tissue damage and produces prostaglandins that manifest pathological effects. It became clear that different NSAIDs had greater or lesser effects on COX-1 when used in therapeutic doses, explaining the variation in side-effects.

The elucidation of the crystal structure of these different enzymes and the skills of medicinal chemists have led to the synthesis of new chemicals with a selectivity for the inducible enzyme, and thus with therapeutic efficacy without those toxic effects resulting from inhibition of the constitutive enzyme. A few compounds, such as meloxicam, etodolac and nimesulide, discovered by empirical screening in rats, also turned out to have selectivity towards COX-2. Interestingly, the focus on COX enzymes has exposed other putative sites for the actions of their prostanoid products, with the consequent possibility of new uses for NSAIDs such as in the prophylaxis or treatment of cancer, preventing pre-term delivery and possibly in treating Alzheimer's disease. The therapeutic value of new selective COX-2 inhibitors, and the pathophysiological significance of COX-1 and COX-2, are reviewed in the following chapters presented by recognized authorities in the field.

John R. Vane
Jack H. Botting

1 Mechanism of action of anti-inflammatory drugs: an overview

J. R. VANE and R. M. BOTTING

Among the many mediators of inflammation, the prostaglandins (PGs) are of great importance. They are released by almost any type of chemical or mechanical stimulus. The key enzyme in their synthesis is prostaglandin endoperoxide synthase (PGHS) or cyclooxygenase (COX) which possesses two catalytic sites. The first, a cyclooxygenase active site, converts arachidonic acid to the endoperoxide PGG_2. The second, a peroxidase active site, then converts the PGG_2 to another endoperoxide PGH_2. PGH_2 is further processed by specific isomerases to form PGs, prostacyclin and thromboxane A_2. Of the PGs, PGE_2 and prostacyclin are the main inflammatory mediators. Cyclooxygenase activity has long been studied in preparations from sheep seminal vesicles and a purified, enzymatically-active COX was isolated in 1976[1]. We now know that COX exists in at least two isoforms, COX-1 and COX-2.

Over 25 years ago, Vane proposed that the mechanism of action of the aspirin-like drugs (non-steroid anti-inflammatory drugs; NSAIDs) was through the inhibition of PG biosynthesis[2] and there is now a general acceptance of the theory. The inhibition by aspirin is due to the irreversible acetylation of the COX site of PGHS, leaving the peroxidase activity of the enzyme unaffected. In contrast to this unique irreversible action of aspirin, other NSAIDs such as ibuprofen or indomethacin produce reversible or irreversible COX inhibition by competing with the substrate, arachidonic acid, for the active site of the enzyme.

The inhibition of PG synthesis by NSAIDs has been demonstrated in a wide variety of systems, ranging from microsomal enzyme preparations, cells and tissues to whole animals and man. For instance, the concentration of PGE_2 is about 20 ng/ml in the synovial fluid of patients with rheumatoid arthritis[3]. This decreases to zero in patients taking aspirin, a good clinical demonstration of the effect of this drug on PG synthesis. Over the last two decades, several new drugs have reached the market based on COX-1 enzyme screens.

Garavito and his colleagues[4] have determined the three dimensional structure of COX-1, providing a new understanding for the actions of COX inhibitors. Each dimer of COX-1 comprises three independent folding units: an epidermal growth factor-like domain, a membrane binding motif and an enzymatic domain. The sites for peroxidase and COX activity are adjacent but spatially distinct. The conformation of the membrane-binding motif strongly suggests that the enzyme integrates into only a single leaflet of the lipid bilayer and is thus a monotopic membrane protein. Three of the helices of the structure form the entrance to the COX channel and their insertion into the membrane could allow arachidonic acid to gain access to the active site from the interior of the bilayer. The COX active site is a long, hydrophobic channel and

Garavito et al.[4] provide evidence to suggest that some of the aspirin-like drugs, such as flurbiprofen, inhibit COX-1 by excluding arachidonate from the upper portion of the channel. Tyrosine 385 and serine 530 are at the apex of the long active site. Aspirin irreversibly inhibits COX-1 by acetylation of the serine 530, thereby excluding access of arachidonic acid to the active site of this enzyme[4]. The S(−) stereoisomer of flurbiprofen interacts via its carboxylate with arginine 120, thereby placing the second phenyl ring within Van der Waal's contact of tyrosine 385. There may be a number of other sub-sites for drug binding in this narrow channel.

The three dimensional structure of COX-2 has also been published[5]. It closely resembles the structure of COX-1, except that the COX-2 active site is slightly larger and can accommodate bigger structures than those which are able to reach the active site of COX-1. A secondary internal pocket of COX-2 contributes significantly to the larger volume of the active site in this enzyme, although the central channel is also bigger by 17%. Although aspirin acetylates Ser 516 in COX-2, this does not prevent an altered metabolism of arachidonic acid to 15(R)-hydroxy-eicosatetraenoic acid [15(R)-HETE]. The conversion to 15-HETE can be inhibited by most NSAIDs including selective COX-2 inhibitors but not by diclofenac or meclofenamic acid[6]. This indicates that an interaction with SER 516 is essential for the inhibitory activity of the fenamates. Selectivity for COX-2 inhibitors can be conferred by replacing His[513] and Ile[523] of COX-1 with Arg and Val respectively. This replacement removes the restriction at the mouth of the secondary side channel and allows access for the more bulky selective COX-2 inhibitors[7].

TWO ISOENZYMES

The constitutive isoform, COX-1, has clear physiological functions. Its activation leads, for instance, to the production of prostacyclin which when released by the endothelium is anti-thrombogenic[8] and when released by the gastric mucosa is cytoprotective[9]. It is also COX-1 in platelets that leads to thromboxane A_2 production, causing aggregation of the platelets to prevent inappropriate bleeding[10]. The existence of the inducible isoform, COX-2, was first suspected when Needleman and his group showed that cytokines induced the expression of COX protein[11] and that bacterial lipopolysaccharide increased the synthesis of PGs in human monocytes in vitro[12] and in mouse peritoneal macrophages in vivo[13]. This increase was inhibited by dexamethasone and associated with de novo synthesis of new COX protein. A year or so later, COX-2 was identified as a distinct isoform encoded by a different gene from COX-1[14–18]. The human COX-2 gene is 8.3 kb in length, similar to the COX-2 gene of mouse and chicken but smaller than the 22 kb human COX-1 gene. The sequence of its cDNA shows 60% homology with the sequence of the noninducible enzyme, with the mRNA for the inducible enzyme being approximately 4.5 kb and that of the constitutive enzyme being 2.8 kb. However, both enzymes have a molecular weight of 71 kDa. The inhibition by the glucocorticoids of the expression of COX-2 is an additional aspect of the anti-inflammatory action of the corticosteroids. The levels of COX-2, normally very low in cells, are tightly controlled by a number of factors including cytokines, intracellular messengers and availability of substrate.

COX-2 is induced by inflammatory stimuli and by cytokines in migratory and other cells, suggesting that the anti-inflammatory actions of NSAIDs are due to the inhibition of COX-2, whereas the unwanted side effects such as damage to the stomach lining and toxic effects on the kidney are due to inhibition of the constitutive enzyme, COX-1[19].

FUNCTIONS OF COX-1 AND COX-2

COX-1 performs a 'housekeeping' function to synthesize PGs which regulate normal cell activity. The concentration of the enzyme largely remains stable, but small (2- to 4-fold) increases in expression can occur in response to stimulation with hormones or growth factors[20,21]. Normally, little or no COX-2 is found in resting cells but its expression can be increased dramatically after exposure of cells to bacterial lipopolysaccharide, phorbol esters, cytokines or growth factors. However, 'constitutive' levels of COX-2 have been detected in some organs such as the brain and the kidney. It is the induction of COX-2 that generates $PGF_{2\alpha}$ to contract the uterus.

The gastrointestinal tract

In most species, including man, the bulk of the protective PGs are synthesized by COX-1, although small quantities of COX-2 can also be expressed in the normal rat stomach[22]. Mice rendered deficient in the gene for COX-1 might be expected to develop spontaneous gastric bleeding or erosions, but they do not[23]. Certainly, there are other 'cytoprotective' mechanisms, such as the synthesis of nitric oxide or CGRP and these might take over in the absence of the PGs.

PGs produced by COX-1 confer protection on the epithelial cells of the crypts of Lieberkühn in the ileum of irradiated mice. Radiation injury results in a decrease in the number of surviving crypt stem cells. These numbers are further reduced by the administration of indomethacin to irradiated mice, but not by administration of a selective COX-2 inhibitor. Since the presence of COX-1 was demonstrated in the epithelial cells of the crypts of non-irradiated mice and in the regenerating crypt epithelium of irradiated animals, PGs produced by COX-1 promote crypt stem cell survival and proliferation[24]. Interestingly, COX-2 mRNA levels are raised in human gastric adenocarcinoma tissues compared to those in normal specimens of gastric mucosal tissue. COX-1 mRNA levels are not elevated in carcinoma[25].

Epidemiological studies have established a strong link between ingestion of aspirin and a reduced risk of developing colon cancer[26,27]. It has also been reported that sulindac causes reduction of PG synthesis and regression of adenomatous polyps which would otherwise develop into rectal carcinomas unless surgically removed[28]. It is interesting that COX-2 is highly expressed in human and animal colon cancer cells as well as in human colorectal adenocarcinomas[29,30]. Human cultured colon cancer (Caco-2) cells transfected with a COX-2 expression vector[31] acquire increased prostaglandin production and invasiveness, reversible with sulindac sulphide. Another human colon cancer cell line, HCA-7, expresses high levels of COX-2 protein constitutively. When HCA-7 cells were implanted as a xenograft in nude mice, tumour formation was inhibited by 90% following treatment with the selective COX-2 inhibitor, SC-58125[32].

Further support for the close connection between COX-2 and colon cancer has come from studies in mice with a mutation of the APC gene. These animals develop a condition similar to familial adenomatous polyposis, characterized by the presence of large numbers of intestinal polyps. However, mice carrying the APC mutation made deficient in the COX-2 gene have very few intestinal polyps, indicating that COX-2 is involved in polyp formation and in neoplasia of the colon. A selective COX-2 inhibitor also reduced the polyposis[33].

The kidney

Maintenance of kidney function is dependent on PGs when the function is compromised in animal models of disease states and also in patients with congestive heart failure, liver cirrhosis or renal insufficiency. Patients are, therefore, at risk of renal ischaemia when PG synthesis is reduced by NSAIDs.

Those kidney cells which synthesize PGs contain mostly COX-1, but low levels of COX-2 mRNA have also been measured[34]. Cultured rat mesangial cells increase production of PGI_2 and PGE_2 after induction of COX-2 with cytokines or growth factors[35]. It is possible that the PGI_2 formed by mesangial cells directly stimulates renin secretion as a feedback control for inhibition of salt reabsorption. Up-regulation of COX-2 expression has been observed in the macula densa following salt deprivation[34].

Mice which lack the gene for production of COX-1 appear healthy and do not show significant signs of kidney pathology. This is in accord with the findings that inhibition of COX-1 by NSAIDs does not alter renal function under normal physiological conditions. However, in COX-2 (-/-) null mice the kidneys fail to continue normal development after birth, and the animals die within 8 weeks of birth[36].

The central nervous system

COX-1 is distributed in neurones throughout the brain but it is most abundant in forebrain, where PGs may be involved in complex integrative functions such as control of the autonomic nervous system, and in sensory processing[37,38]. COX-2 mRNA is induced in brain tissue and in cultured glial cells by pyrogenic substances such as LPS and IL-1[39,40]. However, low levels of COX-2 immunoreactivity and COX-2 mRNA have been detected in neurones of the forebrain without previous stimulation by pro-inflammatory substances[37,38,41]. These 'basal' levels of COX-2 are particularly high in neonates and are probably induced by physiological nervous activity. Intense nerve stimulation leading to seizures induces COX-2 mRNA in discrete neurones of the hippocampus[42], whereas acute stress raises levels in the cerebral cortex[37]. COX-2 mRNA is also constitutively expressed in the spinal cord of normal rats and is likely to be involved with processing of nociceptive stimuli[43].

Fever is produced by an injection of PGE_2 into the preoptic area[44]. Endogenous, fever-producing PGE_2 is thought to originate from COX-2 induced by LPS or IL-1 in endothelial cells lining the cerebral blood vessels[40]. Selective inhibitors of COX-2 such as NS-398 are potent antipyretic agents[45].

The Baltimore Longitudinal Study of Aging, with 1686 participants, reported that the risk of developing Alzheimer's disease is reduced among users of NSAIDs, especially those who have taken the medications for 2 years or more. No decreased risk was evident with paracetamol or aspirin use. However, aspirin was probably taken in a dose too low to have an anti-inflammatory effect. The protective effect of NSAIDs is consistent with evidence of inflammatory activity in the pathophysiology of Alzheimer's disease[46]. Chronic treatment with selective COX-2 inhibitors may therefore slow the progress of Alzheimer's disease without damaging the stomach mucosa[47].

The lungs

Airway hyper-reactivity, a feature of allergic asthma, is associated with inflammation of the airways. Increased expression of COX-2 mRNA and of enzyme protein, with no change in COX-1 levels, has been detected in pulmonary epithelial cells, airway smooth muscle cells, pulmonary endothelial cells and alveolar macrophages treated with LPS or proinflammatory cytokines. In the carrageenin-induced pleurisy model of inflammation, levels of COX-2 protein increased maximally at 2 h in the cell pellets of pleural exudate[48]. This could be accounted for by induction of COX-2 found in all mast cells, in about 65% of resident mononuclear leukocytes and in approximately 8% of extravasated neutrophils present in the exudate[49]. However, lung tissue can also express COX-2 constitutively. COX-2 mRNA was weakly expressed in unstimulated isolated perfused lungs of the rat and this could be up-regulated by nitric oxide (NO) donors[50]. Human lungs obtained from accident victims[51] and cultured human pulmonary epithelial cells expressed more constitutive COX-2 than constitutive COX-1[52,53]. Interestingly, hypoxia induces COX-2 gene expression in isolated, perfused lungs of the rat without affecting levels of mRNA coding for COX-1[50]. This induction of the COX-2 gene by hypoxia was inhibited by NO donors: this may represent one of the mechanisms of the beneficial effect of inhaled NO in pulmonary hypertension. Exposure to environmental pollutants from car exhausts can also induce the COX-2 gene and increase COX-2 protein levels in human, cultured airway epithelial cells, and result in an increased formation of PGE_2 and $PGF_{2\alpha}$[54].

There is good evidence that the leukotrienes, products of 5-lipoxygenase, are important bronchoconstrictors in asthma[55]. Cyclooxygenase products formed by the lung consist mostly of the weak bronchodilator, PGE_2, together with the potent bronchoconstrictor prostanoids, $PGF_{2\alpha}$ and TXA_2. Formation of $PGF_{2\alpha}$ and TXA_2 together with the increased sensitivity to $PGF_{2\alpha}$ in asthmatics may account for a large part of the bronchoconstriction experienced by asthmatic patients. COX-2 is probably up-regulated in the inflamed lungs of asthmatics resulting in increased production of bronchoconstrictor PGs which exert an exaggerated effect on the bronchiolar smooth muscle that has become hyperreactive to constrictor agents. Up-regulation of COX-2 with simultaneous down-regulation of COX-1 by LPS has been reported[56]. Clinical observations in more than 1000 patients have suggested that the selective COX-2 inhibitor, nimesulide, is well tolerated in aspirin-sensitive asthmatics[57]. Aspirin-induced asthma is, therefore, most likely to be associated with inhibition of COX-1. Thus, selective inhibition of COX-2 may provide an additional therapy for asthma.

At the present time, inhaled steroids are the drugs of choice for the treatment of asthma. Part of their beneficial action may be due to down-regulation of the expression of COX-2. Selective COX-2 inhibitors in combination with steroids or with leukotriene antagonists may provide improved treatment for asthmatic patients in the future. Alternatively, the combined COX-2 selective/5-lipoxygenase inhibitors[58] may be the way forward to finding an effective therapy for asthma.

Gestation and parturition

Prostaglandins are important for inducing uterine contractions during labour. NSAIDs such as indomethacin will thus delay premature labour by inhibiting this production of PGs[59]. Furthermore, PG synthesized by COX-1 are apparently essential for the survival of fetuses during parturition, since the majority of offspring born to homozygous COX-1 knock-out mice do not survive[60]: this high mortality of the pups may be due to premature closure of the ductus arteriosus. Expression of COX-1 is much greater than that of COX-2 in fetal hearts, kidneys, lungs and brains as well as in the decidual lining of the uterus[59,61]. Constitutive COX-1 in the amnion could also contribute PGs for the maintenance of a healthy pregnancy[62]. In human amnion cells, COX-1 mRNA is increased by human chorionic gonadotrophin[63].

Female COX-2 knock-out mice are mostly infertile, producing very few offspring due to a reduction in ovulation[64]. Both COX-1 and COX-2 are expressed in the uterine epithelium at different times in early pregnancy and may be important for implantation of the ovum and in the angiogenesis needed for establishment of the placenta[65]. PGs originating from COX-2 may play a role in the birth process since COX-2 mRNA in the amnion and placenta increases markedly immediately before and after the start of labour[61]. It is interesting that $PGF_{2\alpha}$-receptor knock-out mice become pregnant with normal pups, but are unable to give birth[66]: the uterus does not contract at term and does not respond to oxytocin. Thus, oxytocin contracts the mouse uterus by releasing PGs. Glucocorticoids, EGF, IL-1β and IL-4 all stimulate COX-2 production in human amnion cells[67,68] and glucocorticoids can cause premature labour in pregnant sheep, possibly by inducing progesterone-metabolizing enzymes which reduce progesterone levels below those needed to maintain pregnancy[69]. Pre-term labour may be caused by an intra-uterine infection resulting in release of endogenous factors which increase PG production by up-regulating COX-2[68]. Selective inhibitors of COX-2 reduce PG synthesis in fetal membranes and should be useful in delaying premature labour without the side-effects of indomethacin[59].

COX-2/COX-1 INHIBITORY RATIOS OF NSAIDs

Individual NSAIDs show different potencies against COX-1 compared with COX-2 and this nicely explains the variations in the side effects of NSAIDs at their anti-inflammatory doses. Drugs with high potency against COX-2 and therefore a lower COX-2/COX-1 activity ratio, will have anti-inflammatory activity with fewer side effects in the stomach and kidney. Garcia Rodriguez and Jick[70], Langman et al.[71] and Henry et al.[72] have published a comparison of epidemiological data of the gastric side effects of NSAIDs. Piroxicam and indomethacin were amongst those with the highest gastrointestinal toxicity. These drugs have a much higher potency against COX-1 than against COX-2[73]. Thus, when epidemiological results are compared with COX-2/COX-1 ratios, there is a parallel relationship between gastrointestinal side effects and COX-2/COX-1 ratios. COX-2/COX-1 ratios provide a useful comparison of relative values for a series of NSAIDs tested in the same system. However, the COX-2/COX-1 ratio for a particular NSAID will vary according to whether it is measured on intact cells, cell homogenates, purified enzymes or recombinant proteins expressed in bacterial, insect or animal cells. It will also vary when measured in different types of cells derived from various species.

ASSESSMENT OF SELECTIVITY

A number of methods have been described for determining the ED_{50} values for NSAIDs against COX-2 and COX-1, leading to the aforesaid variable values for the COX-2/COX-1 ratio. Table 1 shows values for indomethacin which vary between 0.07[74] and 60[75]. Clearly, cultures of cells from animals (first group) give relatively high values, while microsomal human enzyme preparations (middle group) give a different set. Some of the reasons for variation have been identified. For example, Laneuville et al.[76] added drug and substrate to the human microsomal enzyme at the same time but noted that several NSAIDs, including indomethacin, take 10–20 minutes to produce a full enzyme inhibition. When the drug was incubated for 20 minutes with the enzyme before adding substrate[77] indomethacin was far more potent (especially on COX-2) and the ratio was reduced to 3.5. Other conditions that will lead to variation in results are the absence of protein from the medium and the several hours taken to induce COX-2 in cells.

Some examples of the experimental systems in which COX-2/COX-1 ratios of NSAIDs have been estimated are listed in Table 2. Inhibition of COX-1 is measured

Table 1. Inhibition of COX-1 and COX-2 by indomethacin, determined using different models

Model	COX-2 IC_{50} (μM)	COX-1 IC_{50} (μM)	COX-2/ COX-1 Ratio	References
Cultured animal cells	145	6.6	22	Meade et al. 1993[96]
	1.7	0.028	60	Mitchell et al. 1993[75]
	0.006	0.0002	30	Engelhardt et al. 1996[101]
	0.009	0.0015	6	Klein et al. 1994[97]
Human enzyme preparations	0.97	7.4	1.3	Futaki et al. 1994[98]
	>1000	13	>75	Laneuville et al. 1994[76]
	1.4	0.6	2.3	O'Neill et al. 1994[99]
	0.9	0.1	9	Gierse et al. 1995[100]
	0.35	0.1	3.5	Churchill et al. 1996[77]
Human cells	0.36	0.7	0.51	Patrignani et al. 1994[102]
	0.0012	0.017	~0.07	Grossman et al. 1995[74]
	1.7	0.13	12.5	Young et al. 1996[81]

Table 2. Examples of experimental models used to determine inhibition of COX-1 and COX-2 by NSAIDs

Source of COX-1	Source of COX-2 (LPS or IL-1-stim)	References
Bovine aortic endothelial cells	Mouse macrophages	Mitchell et al., 1993[75]
Guinea pig macrophages	Guinea-pig macrophages	Engelhardt et al., 1996[101]
Human platelets	Rat mesangial cells	Klein et al., 1994[97]
Human gastric mucosa	Human leukocytes	Tavares and Bennett, 1993[80]
Human platelets	Human whole blood	Patrignani et al., 1994[102]
Human whole blood	Human whole blood	Young et al., 1996[81]
Human platelets	Human leukocytes	Grossman et al., 1995[74]
Human enzyme	Human enzyme	Churchill et al., 1996[77]

in unstimulated cells, whereas animal or human cells stimulated with bacterial lipopolysaccharide or interleukin-1 provide a source of COX-2.

Despite these methodological variations the ratios still fall into three broad groups; high ratios for indomethacin, naproxen and piroxicam, approximate equiactivity on the two enzymes for diclofenac and ibuprofen and selectivity for COX-2 for nimesulide, meloxicam, MK-966 and celecoxib. Thus, most of the results published so far support the concept that the unwanted side effects of NSAIDs are due to their ability to inhibit COX-1 whilst their anti-inflammatory (therapeutic effects) are due to inhibition of COX-2. The activities in humans of the highly selective COX-2 inhibitors have now given proof of the concept (see later).

SELECTIVE COX-2 INHIBITION

Meloxicam, nimesulide and etodolac

These NSAIDs were not specifically designed as COX-2 inhibitors and are already available in some countries for the treatment of inflammation. They preferentially inhibit COX-2 rather than COX-1, with a variation in their COX-2/COX-1 ratios of between 0.1 and 0.01.

Meloxicam, which has a 10-fold selectivity towards COX-2 over COX-1 in the human whole blood assay[78], is marketed around the world for use in rheumatoid arthritis and osteoarthritis. In double blind trials in more than 12 000 patients with osteoarthritis and rheumatoid arthritis, meloxicam in doses of 7.5 mg or 15 mg once a day compared in efficacy with standard NSAIDs such as naproxen 750–1000 mg, piroxicam 20 mg and diclofenac 100 mg. Both doses of meloxicam produced significantly fewer gastrointestinal adverse effects than the standard NSAIDs ($p < 0.05$). Discontinuation of treatment due to gastrointestinal side effects was also significantly less frequent with meloxicam (Table 3). Perforations, ulcerations and bleedings occurred in fewer meloxicam-treated patients than in patients treated with piroxicam, diclofenac or naproxen. The frequency of adverse events with meloxicam was significantly less ($p < 0.05$) compared with piroxicam and naproxen[79]. The number of days in hospital for gastrointestinal adverse effects was 124 for diclofenac compared with 5 for meloxicam (Table 3).

Table 3. MELISSA and pharmaco-economy: COX-2 selectivity reduces hospitalizations

	Meloxicam 7.5 mg	Diclofenac 100 mg
No. of patients	4635	4688
Incidence of hospitalizations due to GI adverse events	3(0.06%)	11(0.23%)
Mean duration of hospitalization for GI adverse events (days)	1.7	11.3
Mean duration of stay in ICU for GI adverse events (days)	0	10
Total no. of days in hospital for GI adverse events	5	124
Total no. of days in ICU for GI adverse events	0	50

Nimesulide is currently sold in several European countries and in South America for the relief of pain associated with inflammatory conditions. It is a selective inhibitor of COX-2 with, in human blood assays, some 5- to 20-fold greater potency against this enzyme than against COX-1[78,80,81]. In limited clinical trials for its use in acute and chronic inflammation in patients, it was more effective than placebo and had comparable anti-inflammatory activity to established NSAIDs[82–84]. Epidemiological data suggests that, in long term therapeutic use at anti-inflammatory doses (100 mg twice daily) it causes no more serious gastrointestinal symptoms than placebo[85]. Moreover, nimesulide seems safe to use in aspirin-sensitive asthmatics. In 9 recent studies in over 1000 NSAID-intolerant asthmatic patients there was no cross-reaction with nimesulide at a dose of 100 mg twice a day[57]. At 200 mg twice a day, there were 10 interactions per 100 patients. This could well reflect an activity against COX-1 at the higher dose[57]. A disadvantage of nimesulide is the need for dosing more than once a day because of its relatively short half-life.

Etodolac is marketed in Europe and North America for the treatment of osteoarthritis and rheumatoid arthritis. It has a COX-2/COX-1 ratio of 0.1 on human whole blood[86]. In healthy human volunteers, etodolac twice a day did not suppress gastric mucosal PG production and caused less gastric damage than naproxen[87]. Patients with osteoarthritis or rheumatoid arthritis obtained relief from symptoms equal to other commonly used NSAIDs with etodolac but with a lower incidence of serious gastrointestinal toxicity[88].

Celecoxib and MK-966

These drugs were designed to have high selectivity for COX-2 over COX-1 and are still in clinical development[89,90]. Monsanto/Searle have made inhibitors such as SC 58125, which are some 400-fold more potent in vitro against COX-2 than against COX-1. One of these, celecoxib (SC 58635; Figure 1), is an effective analgesic in humans for moderate to severe pain following tooth extraction[91]. In Phase II trials, patients with osteoarthritis of the knee were treated with twice daily doses of 40 mg, 100 mg or 200 mg. There was significantly greater improvement on all doses than on placebo. The incidence of adverse reactions and withdrawal from the study due to

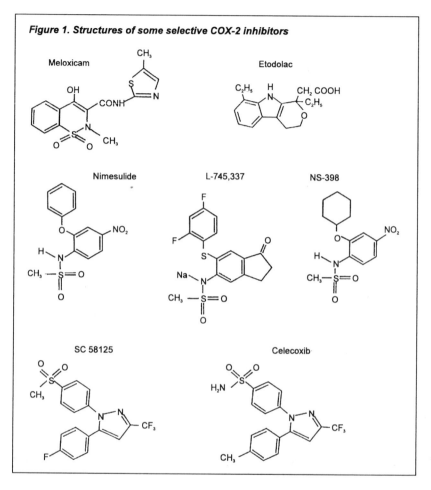

Figure 1. Structures of some selective COX-2 inhibitors

adverse reactions was similar in placebo and celecoxib-treated groups. In a study in patients with rheumatoid arthritis, twice daily doses of 40 mg, 200 mg or 400 mg reduced duration of morning stiffness more than placebo and the number of painful joints was significantly less at the two highest doses than on placebo. No serious adverse events or changes in renal parameters were reported. Celecoxib is currently in Phase III trials in arthritic patients[92].

In whole cell assays, the selective COX-2 inhibitor from Merck-Frosst L-745,337, inhibited COX-2 with an IC_{50} of 20 nM, but was inactive on COX-1 even at doses of 10 µM (COX-2/COX-1 ratio of 1:500)[93]. Another lead compound was the methyl sulphone, L-758,115 (Figure 2), which in whole cells had an IC_{50} for COX-2 of 3.38 µM and for COX-1 of >100 µM, demonstrating a COX-2/COX-1 ratio of less than 0.03. A similar highly selective COX-2 inhibitor from Merck-Frosst, MK-966, is currently undergoing Phase II/III clinical trials. In Phase I studies, a single dose of 250 mg daily for seven days produced no adverse effects on the stomach mucosa, as

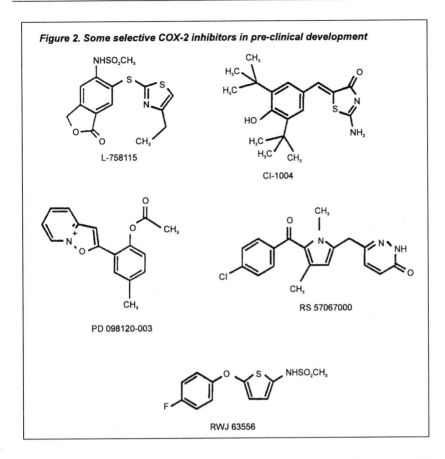

Figure 2. Some selective COX-2 inhibitors in pre-clinical development

evidenced by gastroscopy. After a single dose of 1 g, there was no evidence of COX-1 inhibition in platelets, but activity of COX-2 in LPS-stimulated monocytes *ex vivo* was reduced. For dental pain, MK-966 at 25 mg per dose demonstrated equal analgesic activity to ibuprofen and provided relief from symptoms in a 6-week study of osteoarthritis[94].

Whether or not these new drugs reach the market, their anti-inflammatory effect establishes COX-2 as the inflammatory enzyme. Equally, the lack of gastric side effects establishes that it is inhibition of COX-1 by the other aspirin-like drugs which leads to gastrotoxicity.

New selective COX-2 and dual COX-2/5LO inhibitors

Several pharmaceutical companies have selective COX-2 inhibitors under investigation[58] (Figure 2). Parke-Davis are conducting clinical studies on CI-1004, a combined COX-2 and 5-lipoxygenase inhibitor, which has no gastric toxicity in rats or monkeys and is well tolerated in humans in single doses of up to 100 mg. This drug inhibits recombinant human COX-2 with an IC_{50} of 0.48 µM and has no apparent activity against COX-1. PD 098120-003, another COX-2 inhibitor from Parke-Davis, has no effect on COX-1 and does not cause gastrointestinal toxicity in animals.

RS-57067000, from Roche Bioscience, has a weak effect on COX-1 and does not cause gastric erosions in the rat in doses up to 200 mg/kg. The COX-2/COX-1 ratio for this compound on human recombinant enzymes is less than 0.0006.

Other companies are developing dual COX-2/5-lipoxygenase inhibitors as anti-inflammatory drugs. Johnson and Johnson are evaluating RWJ 63556, which inhibits LTB_4 production in human leukocytes with an IC_{50} of 1 µM and has a COX-2/COX-1 ratio of less than 0.18 determined on human peripheral leukocytes. Procter and Gamble have presented data[58] on PGV 20229 which has no gastrointestinal toxicity in dogs and inhibits leukotriene biosynthesis in RBL-2 cells. The COX-2/COX-1 ratio of PGV 20229 is 0.03 measured on human platelets for COX-1 and on human monocytes for COX-2.

CONCLUSIONS

The fact that the new highly selective inhibitors of COX-2 are analgesic and anti-inflammatory in patients, with no adverse effects on the stomach, gives massive support to the overall concept that inhibition of prostaglandin biosynthesis accounts for the action of aspirin-like drugs. The adverse side effects are due to inhibition of COX-1 whereas the beneficial analgesic, anti-inflammatory and antipyretic effects are due to inhibition of COX-2.

It is estimated that in the USA alone, between 10 000 and 20 000 patients die each year from NSAID-associated toxicity such as perforations and bleeding of the stomach[95]. Clearly, use of the new selective COX-2 inhibitors will reduce this mortality, leading to a new era in the fight against inflammation. If and when the new class of highly selective COX-2 inhibitors reaches the market around the turn of the millennium, deaths from severe gastric toxicity should become a thing of the past.

As well as benefiting arthritic patients, these selective inhibitors may demonstrate new important therapeutic benefits, as anti-cancer agents, preventing premature labour and perhaps even retarding the progression of Alzheimer's disease.

Acknowledgements

The William Harvey Research Institute is supported by grants from Schwarz Pharma Ltd., Servier International Research Institute and Boehringer-Ingelheim.

References

1. Hemler M, Lands WEM, Smith WL. Purification of the cyclooxygenase that forms prostaglandins: Demonstration of two forms of iron in the holoenzyme. J Biol Chem. 1976; 251: 5575–9.
2. Vane JR. Inhibition of prostaglandin synthesis as a mechanism of action for the aspirin-like drugs. Nature. 1971; 231: 232–5.
3. Higgs GA, Vane JR, Hart FD, Wojtulewski JA. Effects of anti-inflammatory drugs on prostaglandins in rheumatoid arthritis. In: Robinson HJ, Vane JR eds. Prostaglandin Synthase Inhibitors. New York, Raven Press; 1974: 165–73.

4. Picot D, Loll PJ, Garavito RM. The x-ray crystal structure of the membrane protein prostaglandin H_2 synthase-1. Nature. 1994; 367: 243–9.
5. Luong C, Miller A, Barnett J, Chow J, Ramesha C, Browner MF. Flexibility of the NSAID binding site in the structure of human cyclooxygenase-2. Nature Struct Biol. 1996; 3: 927–33.
6. Mancini JA, Vickers PJ, O'Neill GP, Boily C, Falgueyret J-P, Riendeau D. Altered sensitivity of aspirin-acetylated prostaglandin G/H synthase-2 to inhibition by nonsteroidal anti-inflammatory drugs. Mol Pharmacol. 1997; 51: 52–60.
7. Wong E, Bayly C, Waterman HL, Riendeau D, Mancini JA. Conversion of prostaglandin G/H synthase-1 into an enzyme sensitive to PGHS-2-selective inhibitors by a double His[513] to Arg and Ile[523] to Val mutation. J Biol Chem. 1997; 272: 9280–6.
8. Moncada S, Gryglewski R, Bunting S, Vane JR. An enzyme isolated from arteries transforms prostaglandin endoperoxides to an unstable substance that inhibits platelet aggregation. Nature. 1976; 263: 663–5.
9. Whittle BJR, Higgs GA, Eakins KE, Moncada S, Vane JR. Selective inhibition of prostaglandin production in inflammatory exudates and gastric mucosa. Nature. 1980; 284: 271–3.
10. Funk CD, Funk LB, Kennedy ME, Pong AS, Fitzgerald GA. Human platelet/erythroleukemia cell prostaglandin G/H synthase: cDNA cloning, expression, and gene chromosomal assignment. FASEB J. 1991; 5: 2304–12.
11. Raz A, Wyche A, Needleman, P. Temporal and pharmacological division of fibroblast cyclooxygenase expression into transcriptional and translational phases. Proc Natl Acad Sci USA. 1989; 86: 1657–61.
12. Fu JY, Masferrer JL, Seibert K, Raz A, Needleman P. The induction and suppression of prostaglandin H_2 synthase (cyclooxygenase) in human monocytes. J Biol Chem. 1990; 265: 16737–40.
13. Masferrer JL, Zweifel BS, Seibert K, Needleman P. Selective regulation of cellular cyclooxygenase by dexamethasone and endotoxin in mice. J Clin Invest. 1990; 86: 1375–9.
14. Xie W, Chipman JG, Robertson DL, Erikson RL, Simmons DL. Expression of a mitogen-responsive gene encoding prostaglandin synthase is regulated by mRNA splicing. Proc Natl Acad Sci USA. 1991; 88: 2692–6.
15. Xie W, Robertson DL, Simmons DL. Mitogen-inducible prostaglandin G/H synthase: A new target for nonsteroidal antiinflammatory drugs. Drug Dev Res. 1992; 25: 249–65.
16. O'Banion MK, Sadowski HB, Winn V, Young DA. A serum- and glucocorticoid-regulated 4-kilobase mRNA encodes a cyclooxygenase-related protein. J Biol Chem. 1991; 266: 23261–7.
17. Kujubu DA, Fletcher BS, Varnum BC, Lim RW, Herschman HR. TIS10, a phorbol ester tumor promoter-inducible mRNA from Swiss 3T3 cells, encodes a novel prostaglandin synthase/cyclooxygenase homologue. J Biol Chem. 1991; 26: 12866–72.
18. Sirois J, Richards JS. Purification and characterisation of a novel, distinct, isoform of prostaglandin endoperoxide synthase induced by human chorionic gonadotropin in granulosa cells of rat preovulatory follicles. J Biol Chem. 1992; 267; 6382–8.
19. Vane J. Towards a better aspirin. Nature. 1994; 367; 215–16.
20. DeWitt DL. Prostaglandin endoperoxide synthase: Regulation of enzyme expression. Biochim Biophys Acta. 1991; 1083: 121–34.
21. Wu KK, Sanduja R, Tsai A-L, Ferhanoglu B, Loose-Mitchell DS. Aspirin inhibits interleukin 1-induced prostaglandin H synthase expression in cultured endothelial cells. Proc Natl Acad Sci USA. 1991; 88: 2384–7.
22. Kargman S, Charleson S, Cartwright M et al. Characterization of prostaglandin G/H synthase 1 and 2 in rat, dog, monkey and human gastrointestinal tracts. Gastroenterology. 1996; 111: 445–54.
23. Langenbach R, Morham SG, Tiano HF et al. Prostaglandin synthase 1 gene disruption in mice reduces arachidonic acid-induced inflammation and indomethacin-induced gastric ulceration. Cell. 1995; 83: 483–92.
24. Cohn SM, Schloemann S, Tessner T, Seibert K, Stenson WF. Crypt stem cell survival in the mouse intestinal epithelium is regulated by prostaglandins synthesized through cyclooxygenase-1. J Clin Invest. 1997; 99: 1367–79.

25. Ristimäki A, Honkanen N, Jänkälä H, Sipponen P, Härkönen M. Expression of cyclooxygenase-2 in human gastric carcinoma. Cancer Res. 1997; 57: 1276–80.
26. Thun MJ, Namboodiri MM, Heath CWJ. Aspirin use and reduced risk of fatal colon cancer. N Engl J Med. 1991; 325: 1593–6.
27. Luk GD. Prevention of gastrointestinal cancer – the potential role of NSAIDs in colorectal cancer. Schweiz Med Wochenschr. 1996; 126; 801–12.
28. Nugent KP, Spigelman AD, Phillips RKS. Tissue prostaglandin levels in familial adenomatous polyposis patients treated with sulindac. Dis Colon Rectum. 1996; 39: 659–62.
29. Kutchera W, Jones DA, Matsunami N et al. Prostaglandin H synthase 2 is expressed abnormally in human colon cancer:Evidence for a transcriptional effect. Proc Natl Acad Sci USA. 1996; 93: 4816–20.
30. Gustafson-Svärd C, Lilja I, Halböök O, Sjödahl R. Cyclooxygenase-1 and cyclooxygenase-2 gene expression in human colorectal adenocarcinomas and in azoxymethane induced colonic tumours in rats. Gut. 1996; 38: 79–84.
31. Tsujii M, Kawako S, DuBois RN. Cyclooxygenase-2 expression in human colon cancer cells increases metastatic potential. Proc Natl Acad Sci USA. 1997; 94: 3336–40.
32. Sheng H, Shao J, Kirkland SC et al. Inhibition of human colon cancer cell growth by selective inhibition of cyclooxygenase-2. J Clin Invest. 1997; 99: 2254–9.
33. Oshima M, Dinchuk JE, Kargman SL et al. Suppression of intestinal polyposis in $Apc^{\Delta716}$ knockout mice by inhibition of cyclooxygenase 2(COX-2). Cell. 1996; 87: 803–9.
34. Harris RC, McKanna JA, Akai Y, Jacobson HR, Dubois RN, Breyer MD. Cyclooxygenase-2 is associated with the macula densa of rat kidney and increases with salt restriction. J Clin Invest. 1994; 94: 2504–10.
35. Nüsing RM, Klein T, Pfeilschifter J, Ullrich V. Effect of cyclic AMP and prostaglandin E_2 on the induction of nitric oxide- and prostanoid-forming pathways in cultured rat mesangial cells. Biochem J. 1996; 313: 617–23.
36. Morham SG, Langenbach R, Loftin CD et al. Prostaglandin synthase 2 gene disruption causes severe renal pathology in the mouse. Cell. 1995; 83: 473–82.
37. Yamagata K, Andreasson KI, Kaufman WE, Barnes CA, Worley PF. Expression of a mitogen-inducible cyclooxygenase in brain neurons; regulation by synaptic activity and glucocorticoids. Neuron. 1993; 11: 371–86.
38. Breder CD, Dewitt D, Kraig RP. Characterization of inducible cyclooxygenase in rat brain. J Comp Neurol. 1995; 355: 296–315.
39. Breder CD, Saper CB. Expression of inducible cyclooxygenase mRNA in the mouse brain after systemic administration of bacterial lipopolysaccharide. Brain Res. 1996; 713: 64–9.
40. Cao C, Matsumura K, Yamagata K, Watanabe Y. Endothelial cells of the brain vasculature express cyclooxygenase-2 mRNA in response to systemic interleukin-1β: a possible site of prostaglandin synthesis responsible for fever. Brain Res. 1996; 733: 263–72.
41. Cao C, Matsumura K, Yamagata K, Watanabe Y. Induction by lipopolysaccharide of cyclooxygenase-2 mRNA in rat brain; its possible role in the febrile response. Brain Res. 1995; 697: 187–96.
42. Marcheselli VL, Bazan NG. Sustained induction of prostaglandin endoperoxide synthase-2 by seizures in hippocampus. J Biol Chem. 1996; 271: 24794–9.
43. Beiche F, Scheuerer S, Brune K, Geisslinger G, Goppelt-Struebe M. Up-regulation of cyclooxygenase-2 mRNA in the rat spinal cord following peripheral inflammation. FEBS Lett. 1996; 390: 165–9.
44. Milton AS. Antipyretic actions of aspirin. In: Vane JR, Botting RM, eds. Aspirin and Other Salicylates. London: Chapman and Hall, 1992: 213–44.
45. Futaki N, Yoshikawa K, Hamasaka Y, Arai I, Higuchi S, Iizuka H, Otomo S. NS-398, a novel non-steroidal anti-inflammatory drug with potent analgesic and antipyretic effects which causes minimal stomach lesions. Gen Pharmacol. 1993; 24: 105–10.
46. Yan SD, Zhu H, Fu J et al. Amyloid-β peptide-receptor for advanced glycation endproduct interaction elicits neuronal expression of macrophage-colony stimulating factor: A proinflammatory pathway in Alzheimer disease. Proc Natl Acad Sci USA. 1997; 94: 5296–301.
47. Stewart WF, Kawas C, Corrada M, Metter EJ. Risk of Alzheimer's disease and duration of NSAID use. Neurology. 1997; 48: 626–32.

48. Tomlinson A, Appleton I, Moore AR et al. Cyclo-oxygenase and nitric oxide synthase isoforms in rat carrageenin-induced pleurisy. Br J Pharmacol. 1994; 113: 693–4.
49. Hatanaka K, Harada Y, Kawamura M, Ogino M, Saito M, Katori M. Cell types expressing COX-2 in rat carrageenin-induced pleurisy. Jap J Pharmacol. 1996; 71(Suppl I): 304P.
50. Chida M, Voelkel NF. Effects of acute and chronic hypoxia on rat lung cyclooxygenase. Am J Physiol 1996; 270: L872–8.
51. O'Neill GP, Ford-Hutchinson AW. Expression of mRNA for cyclooxygenase-1 and cyclooxygenase-2 in human tissues. FEBS Lett. 1993; 330: 156–60.
52. Asano K, Lilly CM, Drazen JM. Prostaglandin G/H synthase-2 is the constitutive and dominant isoform in cultured human lung epithelial cells. Am J Physiol 1996; 271: L126–31.
53. Walenga RW, Kester M, Coroneos E, Butcher S, Dwivedi R, Statt C. Constitutive expression of prostaglandin endoperoxide G/H synthase (PGHS)-2 but not PGHS-1 in human tracheal epithelial cells in vitro. Prostaglandins. 1996; 52: 341–59.
54. Samet JM, Reed W, Ghio AJ et al. Induction of prostaglandin H synthase 2 in human airway epithelial cells exposed to residual oil fly ash. Toxicol Appl Pharmacol. 1996; 141: 159–68.
55. Wenzel SE. Arachidonic acid metabolites: mediators of inflammation in asthma. Pharmacotherapy. 1997; 17 (1 Pt2): 3S–12S.
56. Liu SF, Newton R, Evans TW, Barnes PJ. Differential regulation of cyclo-oxygenase-1 and cyclo-oxygenase-2 gene expression by lipopolysaccharide treatment in vivo in the rat. Clin Sci. 1996; 90: 301–6.
57. Senna GE, Passalacqua G, Andri G et al. Nimesulide in the treatment of patients intolerant of aspirin and other NSAIDs. Drug Safety. 1996; 14: 94–103.
58. Parnham MJ. COX-2 inhibitors at the 8th International Conference of the Inflammation Research Association. Exp Opin Invest Drugs. 1997; 6: 79–82.
59. Bennett P, Slater D. COX-2 expression in labour. In: Vane J, Botting J, Botting R, eds. Improved Non-steroid Anti-inflammatory Drugs. COX-2 Enzyme Inhibitors. Lancaster Kluwer Academic Publishers, and London William Harvey Press, 1996; 167–88.
60. Langenbach R, Morham SG, Tiano HF et al. Prostaglandin synthase 1 gene disruption in mice reduces arachidonic acid-induced inflammation and indomethacin-induced gastric ulceration. Cell. 1995; 83: 483–92.
61. Gibb W, Sun M. Localization of prostaglandin H synthase type 2 protein and mRNA in term human fetal membranes and decidua. J Endocrinol. 1996; 150: 497–503.
62. Trautman MS, Edwin SS, Collmer D, Dudley DJ, Simmons D, Mitchell MD. Prostaglandin H synthase-2 in human gestational tissues: Regulation in amnion. Placenta. 1996; 17: 239–45.
63. Toth P, Li X, Lei ZM, Rao CV. Expression of human chorionic gonadotropin (hCG)/luteinizing hormone receptors and regulation of the cyclooxygenase-1 gene by exogenous hCG in human fetal membranes. J Clin Endocrinol Metab. 1996; 81: 1283–8.
64. Dinchuk JE, Car BD, Focht RJ et al. Renal abnormalities and an altered inflammatory response in mice lacking cyclooxygenase II. Nature. 1995; 378: 406–9.
65. Chakraborty I, Das SK, Wang J, Dey SK. Developmental expression of the cyclo-oxygenase-1 and cyclo-oxygenase-2 genes in the peri-implantation mouse uterus and their differential regulation by the blastocyst and ovarian steroids. J Mol Endocrinol. 1996; 16: 107–22.
66. Narumiya S, Murata T, Hirata M et al. Targeted disruption of genes for the mouse prostanoid receptors. Prost Leuk Essen Fatty Acids. 1996; 55 (Suppl 1): 41.
67. Zakar T, Hirst JJ, Milovic JE, Olson DM. Glucocorticoids stimulate the expression of prostaglandin endoperoxide H synthase-2 in amnion cells. Endocrinology. 1995; 136: 1610–19.
68. Spaziani EP, Lantz ME, Benoit RR, O'Brien WF. The induction of cyclooxygenase-2 (COX-2) in intact human amnion tissue by interleukin-4. Prostaglandins. 1996; 51: 215–23.
69. McLaren WJ, Young IR, Wong MH, Rice GE. Expression of prostaglandin G/H synthase-1 and -2 in ovine amnion and placenta following glucocorticoid-induced labour onset. J Endocrinol. 1996; 151: 125–35.
70. Garcia Rodriguez LA, Jick H. Risk of upper gastrointestinal bleeding and perforation

associated with individual non-steroidal anti-inflammatory drugs. Lancet. 1994; 343: 769–72.

71. Langman MJS, Weil J, Wainwright P et al. Risks of bleeding peptic ulcer associated with individual non-steroidal anti-inflammatory drugs. Lancet. 1994; 343: 1075–8.

72. Henry D, Lim LL-Y, Rodriguez LAG et al. Variability in risk of gastrointestinal complications with individual non-steroidal anti-inflammatory drugs: Results of a collaborative meta-analysis. Br Med J. 1996; 312: 1563–6.

73. Vane JR, Botting RM. New insights into the mode of action of anti-inflammatory drugs. Inflamm Res. 1995; 44: 1–10.

74. Grossman CJ, Wiseman J, Lucas FS, Trevethick MA, Birch PJ. Inhibition of constitutive and inducible cyclooxygenase activity in human platelets and mononuclear cells by NSAIDs and Cox 2 inhibitors. Inflamm Res. 1995; 44: 253–7.

75. Mitchell JA, Akarasereenont P, Thiemermann C, Flower RJ, Vane JR. Selectivity of nonsteroidal antiinflammatory drugs as inhibitors of constitutive and inducible cyclooxygenase. Proc Natl Acad Sci USA. 1993; 90: 11693–7.

76. Laneuville O, Breuer DK, DeWitt DL, Hla T, Funk CD, Smith WL. Differential inhibition of human prostaglandin endoperoxide H synthases-1 and -2 by nonsteroidal anti-inflammatory drugs. J Pharmacol Exp Therap. 1994; 271: 927–34.

77. Churchill L, Graham AG, Shih C-K, Pauletti D, Farina PR, Grob PM. Selective inhibition of human cyclo-oxygenase-2 by meloxicam. Inflammopharmacology. 1996; 4: 125–35.

78. Patrignani P, Panara MR, Sciulli MG, Santini G, Renda G, Patrono C. Differential inhibition of human prostaglandin endoperoxide synthase-1 and -2 by nonsteroidal anti-inflammatory drugs. J Physiol Pharmacol. 1997; 48 (in press).

79. Barner A. Review of clinical trials and benefit/risk ratio of meloxicam. Scand J Rheumatol. 1996; 25 (Suppl 102): 29–37.

80. Tavares IA, Bennett A. Activity of nimesulide on constitutive and inducible prostaglandin cyclo-oxygenase. Int J Tissue React. 1993; 15: 49.

81. Young JM, Panah S, Satchawatcharaphong C, Cheung PS. Human whole blood assays for inhibition of prostaglandin G/H synthases-1 and -2 using A23187 and lipopolysaccharide stimulation of thromboxane B_2 production. Inflamm Res. 1996; 45: 246–53.

82. Weissenbach, R. Clinical trials with nimesulide, a new non-steroid anti-inflammatory agent, in rheumatic pathology. J Int Med Res. 1981; 13: 237–45.

83. Pais JM, Rosteiro FM. Nimesulide in the short-term treatment of the inflammatory process of dental tissues: A double-blind controlled trial against oxyphenbutazone. J Int Med Res. 1983; 11: 149–54.

84. Emami Nouri E. Nimesulide for treatment of acute inflammation of the upper respiratory tract. Clin Ther. 1984; 6: 142–50.

85. Fusetti G, Magni E, Armandola MC. Tolerability of nimesulide. Epidemiological data. Drugs. 1993; 46 (Suppl 1): 277–80.

86. Glaser K, Sung M-L, O'Neill K et al. Etodolac selectively inhibits human prostaglandin G/H synthase 2 (PGHS-2) versus human PGHS-1. Eur J Pharmacol. 1995; 281: 107–11.

87. Laine L, Sloane R, Ferretti M, Cominelli F. A randomised double-blind comparison of placebo, etodolac and naproxen on gastrointestinal injury and prostaglandin production. Gastrointest Endosc. 1995; 42: 428–33.

88. Cummings DM, Amadio P Jr. A review of selected newer nonsteroidal anti-inflammatory drugs. Am Fam Physician. 1994; 49: 1197–202.

89. Seibert K, Zhang Y, Leahy K et al. Pharmacological and biochemical demonstration of the role of cyclooxygenase 2 in inflammation and pain. Proc Natl Acad Sci USA. 1994; 91: 12013–17.

90. Chan C-C, Boyce S, Brideau C et al. Pharmacology of a selective cyclooxygenase-2 inhibitor, L-745,337: a novel nonsteroidal anti-inflammatory agent with an ulcerogenic sparing effect in rat and nonhuman primate stomach. J Pharmacol Exp Ther. 1995; 274: 1531–7.

91. Hubbard RC, Mehlisch DR, Jasper DR, Nugent MJ, Yu S, Isakson PC. SC-58635, a highly selective inhibitor of COX-2, is an effective analgesic in an acute post-surgical pain model. J Invest Med. 1996; 44: 293A.

92. Needleman P. Development of novel COX-2 inhibitors. In: Selective COX-2 Inhibitors:

Pharmacology, Clinical Effects and Therapeutic Potential. Abstracts of the William Harvey Research Conference, Cannes. 1997: 24.

93. Boyce S, Chan C-C, Gordon R et al. L-745,337: a selective inhibitor of cyclooxygenase-2 elicits antinociception but not gastric ulceration in rats. Neuropharmacology. 1994; 33: 1609–11.

94. Ford-Hutchinson A. New highly selective COX-2 inhibitors. In: Selective COX-2 Inhibitors: Pharmacology, Clinical Effects and Therapeutic Potential. Abstracts of the William Harvey Research Conference, Cannes. 1997: 23.

95. Fries J. Toward an understanding of NSAID-related adverse events: the contribution of longitudinal data. Scand J Rheumatol. 1996; 25 (Suppl 102): 3–8.

96. Meade EA, Smith WL, DeWitt DL. Differential inhibition of prostaglandin endoperoxide synthase (cyclooxygenase) isozymes by aspirin and other non-steroidal anti-inflammatory drugs. J Biol Chem. 1993; 268: 6610–14.

97. Klein T, Nüsing RM, Pfeilschifter J, Ullrich V. Selective inhibition of cyclooxygenase 2. Biochem Pharmacol. 1994; 48: 1605–10.

98. Futaki N, Takahashi S, Yokoyama M, Arai S, Higuchi S, Otomo S. NS-398, a new anti-inflammatory agent, selectively inhibits prostaglandin G/H synthase/cyclooxygenase (COX-2) activity in vitro. Prostaglandins. 1994; 47: 55–9.

99. O'Neill GP, Mancini JA, Kargman S et al. Overexpression of human prostaglandin G/H synthase-1 and -2 by recombinant vaccinia virus: inhibition by nonsteroidal anti-inflammatory drugs and biosynthesis of 15-hydroxyeicosatetraenoic acid. Mol Pharmacol. 1994; 45: 245–54.

100. Gierse JK, Hauser SD, Creely DP et al. Expression and selective inhibition of the constitutive and inducible forms of human cyclo-oxygenase. Biochem J. 1995; 305: 479–84.

101. Engelhardt G, Bögel R, Schnitzer C, Utzmann R. Meloxicam: influence on arachidonic acid metabolism. Part 1. *In vitro* findings. Biochem Pharmacol. 1996; 51: 21–8.

102. Patrignani P, Panara MR, Greco A et al. Biochemical and pharmacological characterization of the cyclooxygenase activity of human blood prostaglandin endoperoxide synthases. J Pharmacol Exp Ther. 1994; 271: 1705–12.

2 The structure of human cyclooxygenase-2 and selective inhibitors

M. F. BROWNER

The committed step in the production of prostanoids is the metabolism of arachidonic acid to prostaglandin H_2 (PGH_2) by the enzyme prostaglandin H_2 synthase, also referred to as cyclooxygenase (COX)[1]. Two COX enzymes have been identified[2,3], termed COX-1 and COX-2. The COX-1 protein has been shown to be constitutively expressed in a wide variety of cells, whereas the expression of COX-2 is induced in response to pro-inflammatory stimuli[4]. It is now well established that non-steroidal anti-inflammatory drugs (NSAIDs), such as aspirin, ibuprofen, flurbiprofen and naproxen, block the production of prostaglandins by inhibiting the COX enzymes[5]. More recently, these traditional NSAIDs have been shown to be non-selective, inhibiting both COX-1 and COX-2[6]. A hypothesis derived from these discoveries proposes that the undesirable side effects of classical COX inhibitors results from the inhibition of COX-1, whereas the therapeutic, anti-inflammatory effects result from the inhibition of COX-2[7].

The value of obtaining and utilizing atomic resolution structure information in the drug design and discovery process is now well established and has proven successful for a number of protein targets[8]. The development of selective COX-2 inhibitors is a natural focus for structure-based drug discovery, because atomic resolution pictures of the COX-2 and COX-1 enzymes reveal differences that can be exploited in the design of novel and selective inhibitors. There are, however, several challenges associated with obtaining structures of the COX enzymes, primarily because these enzymes are integral membrane proteins. Success in utilizing a structure-based approach to develop selective COX-2 inhibitors is a first for a membrane-bound protein.

HUMAN COX-2 STRUCTURE

The homodimer structure of human COX-2 was revealed by the X-ray crystal structure (Figure 1)[9]. Protein for the crystallization experiments was obtained from a baculovirus system expressing glycosylated human COX-2 protein that is reconstituted with haem to full activity[10]. The COX-2 homodimer structure is shown in Figure 1. Looking down from the extracellular side of the membrane onto the protein reveals the haem cofactor which is bound in the 'cup-shaped' peroxidase active site of COX-2 (Figure 1a). The peroxidase active site is very much exposed to the extracellular environment. Rotating the protein 180° provides a view from the plane of the membrane, looking up into a channel that is accessed

Figure 1. The structure of human COX-2[9]. The COX-2 homodimer is represented by rendering the secondary structure elements; α-helices are depicted as cylinders, β-strands as thick arrows, connecting loops and turns by ribbons. (a) The view from outside the membrane looking down into the peroxidase active site, which is highly exposed to solvent, reveals the haem cofactor (represented in space-filling mode). (b) Rotating the molecule 180°, top to bottom, provides a view looking up from the plane of the cell membrane past the membrane binding helices, into the cyclooxygenase active site. A selective COX-2 inhibitor is bound at this site (represented in space-filling mode)

(a)

(b)

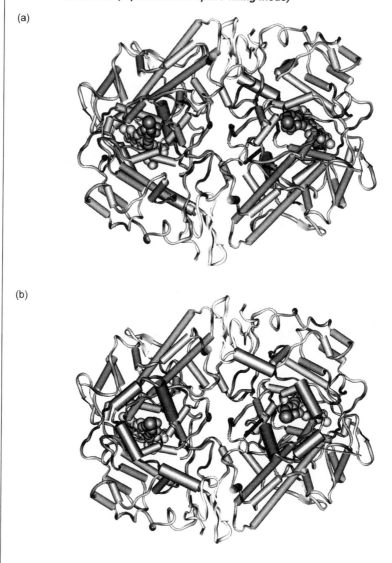

from within the membrane. The COX active site is at the top of this channel. This is also where NSAIDs have been shown to bind in COX-1[11,12] and where selective inhibitors have been shown to bind COX-2[9,13]. Thus reference to the NSAID binding site or the COX active site refers to the same site within the COX enzymes. Extensive contacts between the N-terminal domain of one monomer and the C-terminal domain of the other monomer form the dimer interface and buries approximately 2700 Å^2 of the protein surface. Heterodimers of COX-1 and COX-2 are unlikely to be formed based on amino acid differences at the dimer interface that would create a steric conflict in a COX-1/COX-2 heterodimer[9].

The COX monomer has three distinct domains (Figure 2). The N-terminal domain is a β-sheet domain referred to as the EGF domain because of its similarity to other epidermal growth factor-like protein structures. The next domain, referred to as the membrane binding domain, is composed of four α-helices that bind the protein to the lipid membrane[11] and provide access to the COX active site from within the membrane[9,11]. The third and largest domain is the C-terminal, catalytic domain. The catalytic domain includes both the COX active site and the peroxidase active site with the haem co-factor.

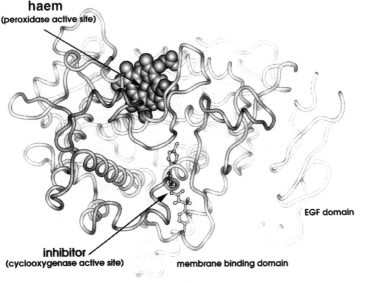

Figure 2. Ribbon diagram of the human COX-2 monomer. The N-terminal EGF domain and the membrane binding domain are labeled. The two active sites contained within the C-terminal catalytic domain are labeled, indicating the haem co-factor in the peroxidase active site and the inhibitor bound at the cyclooxygenase active site

haem
(peroxidase active site)

EGF domain

inhibitor
(cyclooxygenase active site)   membrane binding domain

ENZYME MECHANISM

The COX enzymes possess two distinct enzymatic activities, peroxidase and cyclooxygenase, each associated with an independent active site (Figures 1 and 2). The haem-dependent peroxidase is required for the formation of the tyrosyl radical (Tyr385) which is essential for cyclooxygenase activity[14-17]. The COX reaction inserts two molecules of molecular oxygen into arachidonic acid, producing PGG_2. The X-ray crystal structures of both COX-2 and COX-1 show that Tyr385 is well positioned, at the top of the COX active site on a helix that is the lower boundary of the peroxidase active site, to play a critical role in this mechanism.

The suggestion that the peroxidase active site is directly involved in the final reduction of PGG_2 to PGH_2 requires that the bis-oxygenated substrate move from the COX active site to a binding site near the catalytic residues within the peroxidase active site. Careful examination of the COX-2 structure does not reveal an obvious path by which the oxygenated substrate could move within the enzyme to relocate from the cyclooxygenase active site to the peroxidase active site (Figure 1). Unlike the cyclooxygenase active site, the peroxidase active site is very solvent-exposed, with no well-defined binding pocket for PGG_2. For the peroxidase of COX-2 to be directly involved in the reduction of PGG_2, one needs to envision a mechanism whereby PGG_2 gains selective access to the peroxidase active site from outside the membrane. Based on this information, I favour a mechanism for the generation of the final product that does not directly involve the peroxidase active site. The relatively simple reduction of PGG_2 to PGH_2 could possibly occur in the reducing environment of the membrane.

COMPARISON OF COX-2 AND COX-1

Although the COX-1 and COX-2 proteins are encoded by two different genes[18], the amino acid sequences are closely related. The amino acid sequences of human COX-1 and human COX-2 proteins are 63% identical (78% similar). It is, therefore, not surprising that the overall structure of human COX-2[9] is, in general, very similar to the sheep COX-1 structure[11].

Given the conservation of the catalytic properties of COX-1 and COX-2 it is also not surprising that many of the amino acid residues that define the COX active site (NSAID binding site) are conserved (Figure 3a). In particular, the position and conformation of the amino acid residues Tyr385 at the top of the pocket and Arg120 and Tyr355 at the bottom of the NSAID binding site are virtually identical in the COX-2 and COX-1 structures. Each of these residues has been shown to have important roles in the substrate binding or the enzyme catalysis, based on X-ray crystal structures[9,11,13] and from mutagenesis studies[19,20]. Ser530, which is the site at which the enzyme is acetylated by aspirin, is also conserved in the two isozymes[21,22].

DIFFERENCES AT THE NSAID BINDING SITE

Characterizing the differences between the NSAID binding sites of COX-1 and COX-2 is critical for the utilization of the structure information for drug design (Figure 3).

Figure 3. Comparison of COX-2 and COX-1 NSAID binding sites. (a) Close-up view of the inhibitor binding site in human COX-2 (dark grey ribbon) and sheep COX-1 (light grey) with representative conserved amino acids, Tyr385, Arg120 and Tyr355. The only first shell amino acid difference is shown, residue 523 and two second shell differences are also shown, residues 503 and 513. The COX-1 residue type is in parenthesis. The bound COX-2 inhibitor is represented as a space filling-model[9]. (b) Representation of the accessible molecular surface at the binding site of flurbiprofen in the sheep COX-1 structure (A)[11], and of the inhibitor binding site in human COX-2 (B)[9]. The pictures were generated using the program GRASP[24]

(a)

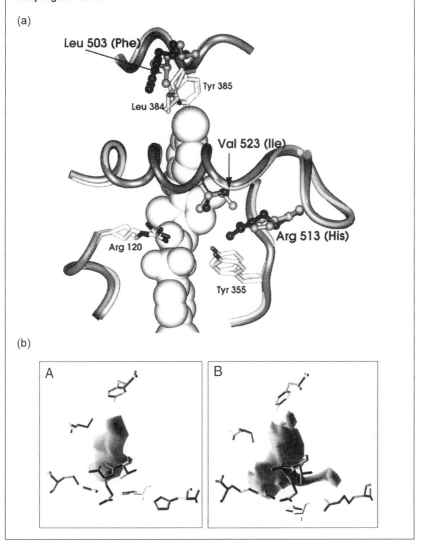

(b)

Amino acid residues surrounding the inhibitor binding site can be defined as belonging to two distinct groups. One group, referred to here as the inner or 'first shell' residues, define the cyclooxygenase active site and are in direct contact with inhibitors bound to either COX-2 or COX-1. The 'second shell' residues also surround the inhibitor binding site, but do not contribute directly to formation of the inhibitor binding site. There are very few amino acid differences between COX-1 and COX-2 in either the first or second shell residues (Figure 3a); however, differences in both sets of amino acids can be exploited for the design of selective inhibitors.

Amino acid residue 523 is the only residue in the first shell, lining the COX active site, that is not identical in COX-2 and COX-1. This amino acid residue is Val in COX-2 and Ile in COX-1. The difference between valine and isoleucine is a single methyl group. The comparison of COX-1 and COX-2 structures revealed that this single amino acid difference creates a second pocket in COX-2 that extends off the inhibitor binding site (Figure 3b). The volume of the COX-2 inhibitor binding site is 25% larger than the NSAID binding site in COX-1, primarily because of the existence of the side pocket[9]. The COX-2 side pocket provides unique access for an inhibitor to reach a second shell amino acid, residue 513. In COX-2 residue 513 is arginine, whereas in COX-1 the residue is histidine. The presence of Arg513 in human COX-2 provides a very good potential hydrogen-binding partner for inhibitors that extend deep into this side pocket. The distinctive shape of the COX-2 NSAID binding site provides a very good starting point for the design of selective inhibitors.

Differences at the top of the NSAID binding site in COX-2 and COX-1 are also observed (Figure 3b). The differences at the top of the inhibitor binding site result from second shell amino acid differences between COX-2 and COX-1. At the top of the inhibitor binding site in COX-1, there is an aromatic residue at position 503 (Phe503) which is in direct contact with a conserved inner shell residue, Leu384 (Figure 3a). In COX-2 residue 503 is the non-aromatic amino acid Leu, which is two methyl groups smaller than Phe. The smaller residue in the second shell of COX-2 (Leu503) does not pack as closely to the conserved first shell residue, Leu384, creating a larger volume at the top of the binding site. The difference in the second shell amino acid residue at position 503 is primarily responsible for size and volume differences in the upper portion of the inhibitor binding site.

SELECTIVE COX-2 INHIBITORS

Differences in the NSAID binding sites of COX-1 and COX-2 revealed by the structures of the two enzymes can be exploited for the design and development of selective COX-2 inhibitors. Information derived from the structure of COX-2 provides a clear rationale for the selectivity of the aryl methyl sulphonamide and sulphonyl compounds, which were originally identified in a screening program[23]. The COX-2 selectivity of these compounds appears to result from the binding of the phenylsulphonamide group into the COX-2 side pocket[13]. We have also shown that very selective COX-2 inhibitors take advantage of the differences at the top of the pocket[9]. The full impact of the structure-based approach on the design of selective

COX-2 inhibitors will become more apparent as compounds developed directly from this information are tested in the clinic.

References

1. Smith WL, Borgeat P, Fitzpatrick FA. The eicosanoids: Cycloxygenase, lipoxygenase, and epoxygenase pathways. In Vance DE, Vance J, eds., Biochemistry of lipids, lipoproteins and membranes. Elsevier Science Publishers; 1991: 297–325.
2. Kujubu DA, Fletcher BS, Varnum BC, Lim RW, Herschman HR. TIS10, a phorbol ester tumor promoter-inducible mRNA from swiss 3T3 cells, encodes a novel prostaglandin synthase/cyclooxygenase. J Biol Chem. 1991; 266: 12866–72.
3. Hla T, Neilson K. Human cyclooxygenase-2 cDNA. Proc Natl Acad Sci USA. 1992; 89: 7384–8.
4. Goppelt-Struebe M. Regulation of Prostaglandin Endoperoxide Synthase (Cyclooxygenase) Isozyme expression. Prostaglandins, Leukotrienes and Essential Fatty Acids. 1995; 52: 213–22.
5. Vane JR. Inhibition of prostaglandin synthesis as a mechanism of action for aspirin-like drugs. Nature New Biol. 1971; 231: 232–5.
6. Mitchell JA, Akarasereenont P, Thiemermann C, Flower RJ, Vane JR. Selectivity of nonsteroidal antiinflammatory drugs as inhibitors of constitutive and inducible cyclooxygenase. Proc Natl Acad Sci USA. 1993; 90: 11693–7.
7. Vane J. Towards a better aspirin. Nature. 1994; 367: 215–16.
8. Verlinde C, Hol W. Structure-based drug design: Progress, results and challenges. Structure. 1994; 2: 577–87.
9. Luong C, Miller A, Barnett J, Chow J, Ramesha C, Browner MF. The structure of human cyclooxygenase-2: Conservation and flexibility of the NSAID binding site. 1996; submitted.
10. Barnett J, Chow J, Ives D et al. Purification, characterization and selective inhibition of human prostaglandin G/H synthase 1 and 2 expressed in the baculovirus system. Biochem Biophys Acta. 1994; 1209: 130–9.
11. Picot D, Loll PJ, Garavito RM. The X-ray crystal structure of the membrane protein prostaglandin H2 synthase-1. Nature. 1994; 367: 243–9.
12. Loll PJ, Picot D, Ekabo O, Garavito RM. Synthesis and use of iodinated nonsteroidal antiinflammatory drug analogs as crystallographic probes of the prostaglandin H_2 cyclooxygenase active site. Biochemistry. 1996; 35: 7330–40.
13. Kurumbail RG, Stevens AM, Gierse JK et al. Structural basis for selective inhibition of cyclooxygenase-2 by anti-inflammatory agents. Nature. 1996; 384: 644–8.
14. Smith WL, Eling TE, Kulmacz RJ, Marnett LJ, Tsai, A. Tyrosyl radicals and their role in hydroperoxide dependent activation and inactivation of prostaglandin endoperoxide synthase. Biochemistry. 1992; 31: 3–7.
15. Tsai A, Kulmacz RJ, Palmer G. Spectroscopic evidence for reaction of prostaglandin H synthase-1 tyrosyl radical with arachidonic acid. J Biol Chem. 1995; 270: 10503–8.
16. Shimokawa T, Kulmacz RJ, Dewitt DL, Smith WL. Tyrosine 385 of prostaglandin endoperoxide synthase is required for cyclooxygenase catalysis. J Biol Chem. 1990; 265: 20073–6.
17. Lassmann G, Odenwaller R, Curtis JF, DeGray JA, Mason RP, Marnett LJ, Eling TE. Electron spin resonance investigation of tyrosyl radicals of prostaglandin H synthase: Relation to enzyme catalysis. J Biol Chem. 1991; 266: 20045–55.
18. Tazawa R, Xu XM, Wu KK, Wang LH. Characterization of the genomic structure, chromosomal location and promoter of human prostaglandin H synthase-2 gene. Biochem Biophys Res Commun. 1994; 203: 190–9.
19. Mancini JA, Riendeau D, Falgueyret, J-P, Vickers PJ, O'Neill GP. Arginine 120 of prostaglandin G/H synthase-1 is required for the inhibition by nonsteroidal anti-inflammatory drugs containing a carboxylic acid moiety. J Biol Chem. 1995; 270: 29372–7.
20. Bhattacharyya DK, Lecomte M, Rieke CJ, Garavito RM, Smith WL. Involvement of arginine 120, glutamate 524, and tyrosine 355 in binding of arachidonate and

2-phenylpropionic acid inhibitors to the cyclooxygenase active site of ovine prostaglandin endoperoxide synthase-1. J Biol Chem. 1996; 271: 2179–84.

21. DeWitt DL, El-Harith EA, Kraemer SA, Andrews MJ, Yao EF, Armstrong RL, Smith WL. The aspirin and heme-binding sites of ovine and murine prostaglandin endoperoxide synthases. J Bio Chem. 1990; 265: 5192–8.

22. Loll PJ, Picot D, Garavito RM. The structural basis of aspirin activity inferred from the crystal structure of inactivated prostaglandin H_2 synthase. Nature Struct Biol. 1995; 2: 637–42.

23. Copeland RA, Williams JM, Giannaras J et al. Mechanism of selective inhibition of the inducible isoform of prostaglandin G/H synthase. Proc Natl Acad Sci USA. 1994; 91: 11202–6.

24. Nicholls A, Sharp K, Honig B. Protein folding and association: insights from the interfacial and thermodynamic properties of hydrocarbons. Proteins. 1991; 11: 281–96.

3 Differential inhibition of COX-1 and COX-2 by NSAIDs: a summary of results obtained using various test systems

M. PAIRET, J. VAN RYN, A. MAUZ, H. SCHIEROK, W. DIEDEREN, D. TÜRCK and G. ENGELHARDT

Since the discovery of a second isoenzyme of cyclooxygenase (COX), COX-2[1,2], it has been hypothesized that the anti-inflammatory effects of non-steroid anti-inflammatory drugs (NSAIDs) are achieved through a mechanism different from that underlying the often seen side-effects of these compounds, including disruption of cytoprotection of the stomach, toxic effects on the kidney and inhibition of platelet aggregation[3]. COX-1 is the constitutive isozyme found under physiological conditions in most tissues, a so-called 'housekeeping' enzyme, while COX-2 expression is induced, particularly during inflammatory processes[4]. It has been proposed that COX-2 inhibition is the relevant target for the anti-inflammatory effects of NSAIDs, whereas inhibition of COX-1 is responsible for their gastric and renal side-effects[3,4]. Most available NSAIDs block both COX-1 and COX-2 to a similar degree; however, newer compounds with selective inhibition of COX-2 should retain the anti-inflammatory activity of NSAIDs but have minimal gastro-intestinal side-effects.

A large number of in vitro assays have been developed to characterize the COX-1 and COX-2 inhibitory activities of NSAIDs. The inhibitory activities are expressed as IC_{50} values (the concentration at which 50% of the activity is inhibited), the index of selectivity is expressed as the ratio of the IC_{50} values for COX-2 and for COX-1. The various test systems developed have produced a multitude of IC_{50} values and ratios and thus given rise to confusing comparisons.

This chapter aims to provide a critical analysis of the in vitro test systems available. In addition, the in vivo relevance of in vitro findings will also be analysed. When results are given, they will be expressed as IC_{50} values and $IC_{50}COX-2/IC_{50}COX-1$ ratios. Under these conditions, low ratios indicate a preferential inhibition of COX-2. It should be stressed, however, that strictly speaking such ratios can only be calculated when the concentration-response curves are parallel. In practice, this condition is not always confirmed. Thus, the COX-2/COX-1 ratios can only be considered as estimates.

It should also be stressed that, due to the time-dependency of COX-2 inhibition, the indices of selectivity obtained result not only from the initial binding of the NSAIDs to the enzymes but also (and most importantly) from the incubation time and type of time-dependency of COX-2 inhibition.

IN VITRO TEST SYSTEMS

The in vitro systems most commonly used to test for COX-2 selectivity are listed in Table 1. Depending on the test system, the experimental conditions may vary greatly. The different experimental conditions may include: the source of enzymes (human or animal), the cell system used (intact normal cells, cell lines or transfected cells), the method of enzyme preparation (purified enzymes, microsomal or whole cell assays), the COX-2 inducing agent (lipopolysaccharide (LPS), interleukin-1 (IL-1) or another cytokine). In addition, other differences can include the source of arachidonic acid as substrate and its concentration, the incubation time with drug, with the COX-2 inducing agent or with arachidonic acid, and the protein concentration in the medium.

Table 1. In vitro assays most commonly used to characterize the COX-1 and COX-2 inhibitory activities of NSAIDs

COX-1	COX-2
Ram seminal vesicle	Sheep placenta
Bovine aortic endothelial cells	LPS-stimulated mouse macrophages
Human washed platelets	IL-1 stimulated rat mesangial cells
Unstimulated guinea pig macrophages	LPS-stimulated guinea pig macrophages
Mouse recombinant enzyme	Mouse recombinant enzyme
Human cell lines: ex: histiocytic lymphoma cells U-937	Human cell lines. ex: osteosarcoma cell line 143.98.2
Human recombinant enzyme: purified enzyme/microsomes/homogenates/whole cell assay	Human recombinant enzyme: purified enzyme/microsomes/homogenates/whole cell assay
Human gastric mucosa pieces	LPS-stimulated human monocytes
Isolated human platelets	LPS-stimulated human monocytes
Clotting human whole blood	LPS-stimulated human whole blood

Ram seminal vesicle vs sheep placenta

From a historical point of view, seminal vesicle is the tissue where prostaglandin synthesis was discovered[5,6]. As early as 1988, it was noted that in spite of treatment with antibodies raised against COX purified from ram seminal vesicle (now known to be COX-1), fibroblasts were still able to increase their prostaglandin biosynthetic activity in response to IL-1, suggesting the existence of an inducible COX[7]. This hypothesis was supported by studies in the field of reproductive biology. Hormonal induction was demonstrated in ovaries and in human amnion, demonstrating a role for this isoform in the induction of ovulation[8] and parturition[9]. It is therefore not surprising that one of the first test systems developed for characterizing COX-1 and COX-2 activities used ram seminal vesicle and sheep placenta. The main drawbacks of this model are that animal instead of human material is used and that purified enzymes are used instead of whole cells. Furthermore, the selected organs are not target organs for the anti-inflammatory and side-effects of NSAIDs. In addition, inhibition of COX-2 activity from sheep placenta is highly dependent on the experimental conditions, particularly the incubation time with the drug and concentration of arachidonic acid. Subtle variations in the experimental conditions may lead to significant differences in the IC_{50} values and selectivity ratios. Nevertheless, this test system has been successfully used to characterize preferential or selective COX-2 inhibitors such as NS-398[10], meloxicam[11], nimesulide[12] and flosulide[13,14].

Bovine aortic endothelial cells vs LPS-stimulated mouse macrophages

This model was used in the first study comparing the differential inhibition of COX-1 and COX-2 by various NSAIDs[15]. An advantage of this model is that the same incubation times with drug and arachidonic acid are used for both COX-1 and COX-2. This is particularly important because of the time-dependency of COX-2 inhibition. The main drawback is that animal cells are used instead of human cells. When results obtained in this model are compared with those obtained in other test systems using human material, the rank order for COX-2 selectivity looks representative, with only a few exceptions. This model, however, tends to overestimate the effect of oxicams on COX-1, as indicated by a COX-2/COX-1 ratio of 250 for piroxicam[16], 15 for ibuprofen[15], 0.8 for meloxicam[16] and 0.7 for diclofenac[15]. In addition, it also tends to underestimate the effects of naproxen on COX-1 (ratio 0.6)[15].

Human washed platelets vs IL-1 stimulated rat mesangial cells

Human platelets have been demonstrated in many studies to express exclusively COX-1. COX-2 can be induced by IL-1β in mesangial cells, which have macrophage-like functions in the kidney. Human platelets and IL-1β-stimulated rat mesangial cells were therefore used to characterize the COX-2 selectivity of flosulide[17]. The main drawback of this model is that cells originating from two different species are used. Furthermore, this test system seems to be more sensitive for COX-2 than for COX-1 inhibition as indicated by a COX-2/COX-1 ratio of 0.07 for diclofenac. Nevertheless, the rank order for COX-2 selectivity of the compounds tested looks representative (flosulide > diclofenac > indomethacin).

Unstimulated vs LPS-stimulated guinea pig macrophages

This model was used in one of the first studies comparing the differential inhibition of COX-1 and COX-2 by various NSAIDs. Unstimulated guinea pig macrophages were used to test for COX-1 activity and guinea pig macrophages stimulated by LPS were used to test for COX-2 activity. An advantage of this model is that intact cells are used and that the same cell types and the same incubation times are used for both COX-1 and COX-2. A drawback is that animal cells instead of human cells are used. Furthermore, no highly selective inhibitors were tested, the most selective compound for COX-2 in this model was meloxicam with a COX-2/COX-1 ratio of 0.3[18].

Mouse recombinant enzymes

The advantage of using recombinant enzymes is that the same expression systems and the same incubation times are used for both COX-1 and COX-2. No induction phase is required since COX-2 is constitutively expressed by the transfected cells. A main drawback is that mouse instead of human enzymes are used. Furthermore, penetration and distribution of the drug into the cell is not taken into account, since cell homogenates or microsomal preparations but not whole cell assays are used. There is also a large heterogeneity in the protein concentration in this model when performed in different laboratories. This is a critical issue when testing compounds such as NSAIDs which are known to bind strongly to plasma proteins.

Taken as a whole, the results obtained using mouse recombinant enzymes look representative. Standard NSAIDs are more active on COX-1 than on COX-2, nimesulide is slightly more potent on COX-2 than on COX-1 and NS-398 and SC-58125 are clearly COX-2 selective[19-21]. One confusing result was the low ratio of 6-MNA, the active metabolite of nabumetone, suggesting a COX-2 selectivity, which could not be confirmed in several other test systems.

Human cell lines

Various human cell lines have been used, including histiocytic lymphoma cells U-937 and megakaryocytic cell line DAMI for COX-1 activity, and osteosarcoma cell line 143.98.2 and monocytic cell line Mono Mac 6 for COX-2 activity[22,23]. An advantage with cell lines is that human 'whole' cells are used. Drawbacks are that immortalized cells may be very different from normal cells regarding, for example, drug penetration and distribution. This test system seems to be more sensitive for COX-2 than for COX-1 inhibition, as indicated by COX-2/COX-1 ratios of ~0.1 for standard NSAIDs such as sulindac, ibuprofen and diclofenac and very low ratios for preferential and selective COX-2 inhibitors. This assay system is normally used for screening purposes only.

Human recombinant enzymes

Various assays with human recombinant enzymes have been described, including whole cell assays, microsomal preparations, cell homogenates and purified enzymes[24-32]. The advantages of such models are that human enzymes are utilized and that the same expression systems are used for both COX-1 and COX-2. However, when microsomes, cell homogenates and purified enzymes are used, penetration and distribution of the drug into the cell is not taken into account. Furthermore, immortalized transfected cells used in whole cell assays may have different properties to 'normal' cells. It should be noted that the experimental conditions also vary between laboratories. These differences are summarized in Table 2 and include: (1) the gene expression system used for gene replication, (2) the cell line transfected with the COX-1 or COX-2 gene, (3) the pre-incubation time with the drug, (4) the concentration of and the incubation time with arachidonic acid, and (5) the assay components (purified enzymes, homogenates, microsomes or whole cells). Studies with purified enzymes were aimed at investigating the time-dependency of COX-2 inhibition rather than the COX-2 selectivity of various compounds[24,25]. They will not be discussed here, instead only studies with microsomal preparations or homogenates and whole cells are presented.

Results obtained using microsomal assays by three independent laboratories are summarized in Table 3. The IC_{50} values vary greatly between laboratories, for example from 0.013 to 0.60 μM for indomethacin and from 0.015 to 0.12 for diclofenac on COX-1. These differences may be related to different protein concentrations in the medium. However, the COX-2/COX-1 ratios seem to be reproducible between the laboratories: 2.3, 5.7 and 3.5 for indomethacin or 0.8, 1.5 and 0.5 for diclofenac. No

Table 2. Different experimental conditions in assays using human recombinant enzymes

	Expression system	Transfected cell line	Pre-incubation with drug	Incubation with arachidonic acid	Assay
Barnett[24] (Copeland[25])	Baculovirus	Sf9 insect cells	Variable	2 min, 50 µM	Purified enzymes
Gierse[29]	Baculovirus	Sf21 insect cells	10 min	10 min, 10 µM	Homogenates
Laneuville[26]	Simian virus SV40	COS-1 cells	Instantaneous	Instantaneous, 10 µM	Microsomes
O'Neil[27]	Vaccinia virus	COS-7 cells	5 min	40 min, 2 µM	Microsomes
Glaser[28]	Baculovirus	Sf9 insect cells	30 min	35 sec, 30 µM	Microsomes
Churchill[30]	Baculovirus	Sf9 insect cells	20 min	20 min, 2 µM	Microsomes
Churchill[30]	pCR/CMV	COS A.2 cells	30 min	60 min, 30 µM	Whole cell
Cromlish[31]	Baculovirus	Sf9 insect cells	15 min	10 min, 10 µM	Whole cell
Kargman[32]	pEE14	CHO cells	15 min	15 min, 10 µM	Whole cell

Table 3. Differential inhibition of COX-1 and COX-2 by various NSAIDs using human recombinant enzymes in microsomal assays or cell homogenates. IC_{50} values are expressed in µmol/l. Ratios given are the ratio of the IC_{50} of COX-2/IC_{50} of COX-1. These ratios were not given in Refs 27, 29, 30. 6-MNA is the active metabolite of nabumetone. +, > 20% inhibition at 300 µM

	O'Neill et al.[27]			Glaser et al.[28]			Churchill et al.[30]			Gierse et al.[29]		
	IC_{50} COX-1	IC_{50} COX-2	Ratio	IC_{50} COX-1	IC_{50} COX-2	Ratio	IC_{50} COX-1	IC_{50} COX-2	Ratio	IC_{50} COX-1	IC_{50} COX-2	Ratio
Indomethacin	0.60	1.4	2.3	0.013	0.074	5.7	0.10	0.35	3.5	0.1	0.2	2
Naproxen	300	>300	>1	1.6	21	13.1	2.7	~50	18.5	1.1	36	33
Piroxicam	60	>300	>5							13	100	>7
Ibuprofen										3.3	37.5	11.4
Tenidap				1.6	3.1	1.9	13.88	~80	5.8			
6-MNA				NA	NA		~100	NA+	>3			
Sulindac sulfide	5.2	10.7	2.1									
Meclofen. acid	0.28	0.10	0.4									
Diclofenac	0.12	0.10	0.8	0.015	0.022	1.5	0.059	0.031	0.5			
Nimesulide							~50	9.4	0.2			
Etodolac				1.5	1.4	0.09						
Meloxicam							36.6	0.49	0.01			

highly selective COX-2 inhibitor was tested. However, a preferential inhibition of COX-2 was found for compounds such as meloxicam, etodolac and nimesulide. Results obtained using cell homogenates are roughly similar to those obtained using microsomal preparations (Table 3).

Results obtained in a whole cell assay in three different publications are summarized in Table 4. These results appear reproducible between different laboratories. Standard NSAIDs are equipotent on COX-1 and COX-2 or inhibit COX-1 preferentially. Among standard NSAIDs, diclofenac and piroxicam seem to have the most favourable ratios. This finding is in agreement with results obtained using other test systems for diclofenac but not for piroxicam. A preferential inhibition of COX-2 is found for nimesulide and meloxicam. Compounds such as flosulide, DuP-697, NS-398 and L-745,337 are highly selective for COX-2. It should be stressed that only the IC_{50} values were given in the original publications, not the COX-2/COX-1 ratios which are only given as rough estimates in Table 4.

Human gastric mucosa pieces vs LPS-stimulated human monocytes

In an attempt to represent the clinical situation more closely, human gastric pieces and LPS-stimulated human leucocytes have been used to test for COX-1 and COX-2 activity, respectively[33,34]. A drawback of this model is that the incubation times are different for COX-1 (30 minutes) and COX-2 (24 hours). As a consequence, testing pro-drugs may overestimate COX-2 inhibitory activity[33]. In addition, the absence of proteins in the leucocyte assay also tends to overestimate COX-2 inhibitory activity of test compounds. In fact, from the data published, no IC_{50} for COX-2 inhibition could be calculated since even the lowest concentrations tested inhibited enzyme activity by more than 70%. Nevertheless, this model indicates future trends in the development of in vitro test systems, by combining assays with cell types which are target cells for the therapeutic and main side-effects of NSAIDs.

Isolated human platelets vs LPS-stimulated human monocytes

The advantage of such a model is that 'normal' human cells are used[35]. A drawback is that no protein is added to the medium and, consequently, drug binding to proteins cannot be taken into account. Furthermore, the results obtained do not appear representative. When they are compared with those obtained with the same compounds in a whole blood assay, which also uses platelets for COX-1 activity and LPS-stimulated monocytes for COX-2 activity, but in the presence of plasma, significant differences are found. All NSAIDs tested were more active on COX-2 than on COX-1 when using isolated cells without proteins. Indomethacin and sulindac had a high selectivity for COX-2 and diclofenac was even more selective for COX-2 than the standard selective COX-2 inhibitors, flosulide and NS-398.

Human whole blood assay

This test system uses clotting human whole blood to test for COX-1 activity and whole blood stimulated by LPS to test for COX-2 activity. Depending on the study, the experimental conditions may vary. The most relevant differences for COX-1 are

Table 4. Differential inhibition of COX-1 and COX-2 by various NSAIDs using human recombinant enzymes in whole cell assays. IC_{50} values are expressed in μmol/l. Ratios given are the ratio of the IC_{50} of COX-2/IC_{50} of COX-1. All ratios were not given in the original publications. 6-MNA is the active metabolite of nabumetone. The lowest IC_{50} values from Ref. 32 are presented here

	Churchill et al.[30]			Cromlish et al.[31]			Kargman et al.[32]		
	IC_{50} COX-1	IC_{50} COX-2	Ratio	IC_{50} COX-1	IC_{50} COX-2	Ratio	IC_{50} COX-1	IC_{50} COX-2	Ratio
Aspirin	4.70	16.03	3.4	0.0015	0.12	82	14.9	5–70	~1
Ketoprofen				0.0008	0.069	87	0.001	0.002	2
Flurbiprofen	0.019	0.030	1.6	0.0019	0.052	27	0.013	0.016	1.2
Indomethacin	0.33	7.08	21	0.45	6.3	14			
Naproxen	2.03	0.98	0.5	0.8	0.53	0.7			
Piroxicam				2.9	>50	17			
Ibuprofen	2.26	15.72	7				0.472	0.465	1
6-MNA	8.40	>300	>36						
Sulindac sulphide				0.006	0.29	4.8			
Diclofenac	0.0026	0.001	0.4	0.003	0.006	2	0.005	0.001	0.2
Nimesulide	1.61	0.36	0.2	5.2	0.87	0.16			
Meloxicam	2.24	0.16	0.07						
Flosulide				>18	0.02	0.001			
DuP-697							0.041	0.002	0.05
NS-398				7.7	0.004	0.0005	0.864	0.003	0.003
L-745,337				>93	0.26	0.003	47.6	0.02	0.0004

that whole blood may or may not be pre-incubated with the drug and that clotting is either spontaneous or induced. For COX-2, different concentrations of LPS are used and the incubation time with LPS and with the drug may vary from 5 to 24 hours. Furthermore, aspirin is sometimes added to block any residual COX-1 activity. The different experimental conditions are summarized in Table 5.

The human whole blood assay has many advantages. First, intact human cells are used which are target cells for the anti-inflammatory effects (monocytes) and the side-effects (platelets) of NSAIDs. Second, plasma proteins present in whole blood allow a better representation of in vivo interactions in the presence of NSAIDs. Third, whole blood used for both assays is taken from the same volunteer (or patient) at the same time to allow a direct comparison of the results from each assay. Fourth, the assay can be performed using blood from volunteers (or patients) who have previously been treated with NSAIDs (ex vivo assay) thus allowing a comparison of the in vivo relevance of in vitro findings. The main drawback is that different incubation times are used for COX-1 and COX-2, since COX-2 has to be induced. In addition, cell types other than platelets and monocytes, such as gastric mucosa cells and synoviocytes would be more representative target cells for measuring the beneficial and detrimental effects of NSAIDs.

Results obtained by different laboratories, including ours, using the human whole blood assay are summarized in Table 6. IC_{50} values and COX-2/COX-1 ratios are reproducible between laboratories with only a few exceptions, such as naproxen (ratio varies between 0.4[38] and 9.5[39]). Standard NSAIDs are roughly equipotent on both isoenzymes, meloxicam and nimesulide in two studies and etodolac in one study are preferential inhibitors of COX-2, flosulide, DuP-697, NS-398, L-745,337 and SC 58125 are selective for COX-2.

ANALYSIS OF RESULTS OBTAINED IN VARIOUS TEST SYSTEMS

It is apparent that many different in vitro test systems are available and, depending on the test system used, different IC_{50} values and COX-2/COX-1 ratios are obtained. As a consequence, comparisons of IC_{50} values and ratios obtained with different compounds can only be performed when the compounds were tested in the same system. Furthermore, the value of each test system should be taken into account when analysing results. For example results obtained in a human whole blood assay are probably more representative than results obtained using animal enzymes in an artificial milieu. Preferential/selective inhibition of COX-2 can only be determined when comparative data are available from several representative models. Comparing results from different compounds obtained from different models leads to confusing results[40,41] and should not be done. In addition, IC_{50} values obtained in vitro should not be compared with plasma concentrations, since in most cases drug binding to plasma proteins is not taken into account in vitro. One exception to this rule may be the human whole blood assay, since plasma proteins present in whole blood may allow a good representation of in vivo interactions in the presence of NSAIDs.

The analysis of the results obtained with different compounds in different test

Table 5. Different experimental conditions used in the human whole blood assay

	Patrignani et al [36,37]	Glaser et al [28]	Young et al [38]	Brideau et al [39]
COX-1: Clotting whole blood				
pre-incubation	No	4 hr 45 min	4 hr 30 min	No
clotting induced?	spontaneous	A23187 (30 min)	A23187 (30 min)	spontaneous
clotting time	1 hr	30 min	30 min	1 hr
incubation	1 hr	30 min	30 min	1 hr
assay	TxB$_2$	TxB$_2$	TxB$_2$	TxB$_2$
COX-2: LPS-stimulated whole blood				
pre-incubation	No	15 min	No	15 min
stimulation with LPS	10 µg/ml, 24 hr (4 hr)	5 µg/ml 5 hr	10 µg/ml 5 hr	100 µg/ml 24 hr
incubation	24 hr	5 hr	5 hr	24 hr
± aspirin?	– (+)	–	– (+)	–
assay	PGE$_2$	TxB$_2$	TxB$_2$	PGE$_2$

Table 6. Differential inhibition of COX-1 and COX-2 (IC_{50}) by various NSAIDs in the human whole blood assay. IC_{50} values are expressed in µmol/l. Ratio describes the ratio of the IC_{50} of COX-2/IC_{50} of COX-1

	Patrignani et al[37]			Brideau et al[39]			Young et al[38]			Glaser et al[28]			Pairet et al		
	COX-1	COX-2	Ratio	COX-1	COX-2	Ratio	COX-1	COX-2	Ratio	COX-1	COX-2	Ratio	COX-1	COX-2	Ratio
ASA							2.8	>167	>59						
Flurbiprofen	0.9	0.9	1.0	0.44	6.42	14	0.55	7	13						
Naproxen	15.6	27.8	1.8	7.76	73.74	9.5	11.0	4.3	0.4	20	23	1.2			
Ibuprofen	9.2	18.3	2.0	4.75	>30	>6	9.2	56	6.1						
Piroxicam	2.86	0.93	0.3	0.76	8.99	12	2.8	7.3	2.6						
Indomethacin	0.53	0.28	0.5	0.16	0.46	2.9	0.13	1.7	13				0.17	0.14	0.8
6-MNA	278	187	0.7	ND	>30		83	301	3.6						
Diclofenac				0.14	0.05	0.4	0.17	0.12	0.7						
Nimesulide	9.2	0.52	0.06				17	3.2	0.2	34	3.4	0.1			
Etodolac															
Meloxicam	4.8	0.43	0.09										3.27	0.25	0.08
Flosulide				32.3	0.75	0.02									
DuP-697				1.18	0.06	0.05									
NS-398	16.8	0.10	0.006	4.81	0.47	0.09	11	0.3	0.03						
L-745,337	369	1.5	0.004	>30	9.67	<0.3									
SC58125	38.7	0.27	0.007	>30	2.25	<0.08							20	<0.48	<0.02

systems indicates the following trends: (1) Standard NSAIDs are either equally effective on COX-1 and COX-2, or slightly more active on COX-1 than on COX-2. Among standard NSAIDs, diclofenac seems to have the most favourable profile. (2) Meloxicam and nimesulide inhibit COX-2 preferentially but not exclusively and some COX-1 inhibitory activity was present in several test systems. Furthermore, preferential inhibition of COX-2 was also shown for etodolac in two models. (3) Developmental compounds or pharmacological tools such as flosulide, DuP-697, NS-398, SC 58125 and L-745,337 inhibit COX-2 selectively.

IN VIVO RELEVANCE OF IN VITRO FINDINGS

The in vivo relevance of in vitro findings should be carefully analysed. This point is particularly important for compounds with a 'relative' selectivity, such as meloxicam, nimesulide and etodolac. Therapeutic concentrations may be compared with the effective concentrations in a human whole blood assay in vitro, as a first approach. However, as soon as in vivo results are available, such comparisons will be superseded by the experimental data obtained in vivo. Figure 1 illustrates the concentration–response curves for inhibition of COX-1 and COX-2 by meloxicam in a human whole blood assay in vitro. In addition, the therapeutic concentrations at steady state are also indicated for the 7.5 mg/day and 15 mg/day doses (Figure 1A and 1B, respectively). All concentrations (in vitro and in vivo) are given in $\mu g/ml$ whole blood. From this analysis, it would be expected that meloxicam, 7.5 mg/day, inhibits COX-2 by 55–75% and COX-1 by ~10%. With 15 mg/day, an inhibition of COX-2 by 80–90% accompanied by a 15–30% inhibition of COX-1 would be expected.

According to this model, it would appear that compounds with a relative selectivity for COX-2, such as meloxicam, require a flat plasma concentration curve to maintain levels above the effective inhibitory concentration for COX-2 but below the effective inhibitory concentration for COX-1. Figure 2 shows drug concentrations in whole blood with 7.5 and 15 mg/day meloxicam (Figure 2A and 2B, respectively). Concentrations in whole blood were calculated from plasma concentrations, assuming that drug concentrations in red cells are negligible and a haematocrit of 45%. IC_{50} values for COX-1 and COX-2 inhibition are also indicated. All concentrations (in vitro and in vivo) are given in $\mu g/ml$ whole blood. When similar simulations are performed for nimesulide at the recommended doses of 100 and 200 mg given twice daily, some inhibition of COX-1 is expected with 100 mg and a significant inhibition (>50%) should occur with 200 mg (Figure 3).

The differential inhibition of COX-1 and COX-2 by NSAIDs in vivo is classically performed by investigating the effects of repeated administration of anti-inflammatory doses in humans, by using a whole blood assay ex vivo, or on markers of COX-1 activity such as platelet aggregation, serum thromboxane B_2 (TxB_2) or urinary excretion of PGE_2 (this last parameter can only be measured in females). A human pharmacology study compared the effects of 7.5 mg/day meloxican with 25 mg indomethacin given three times per day on platelet aggregation, serum TxB_2 and urinary excretion of PGE_2 in human female volunteers[45]. Platelet aggregation and TxB_2 were almost completely blocked by indomethacin and urinary excretion of PGE_2

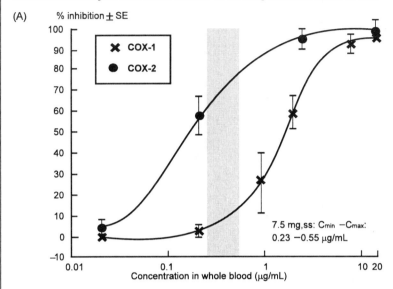

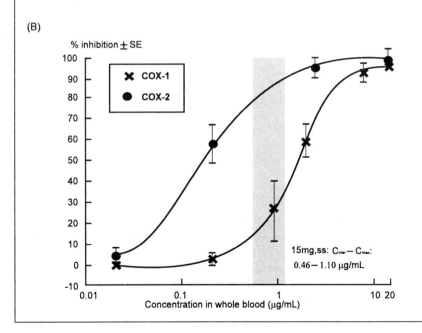

Figure 1. Comparison of concentration–response curves for COX-1 and COX-2 inhibition by meloxicam with therapeutic concentrations at the recommended doses of 7.5 (A) and 15 (B) mg/day. Data were taken from Ref. 37 for the human whole blood assay in vitro and from Ref. 42 for drug concentrations in vivo

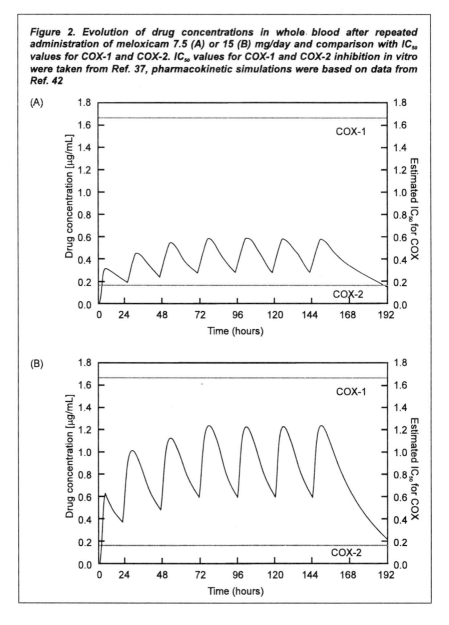

Figure 2. Evolution of drug concentrations in whole blood after repeated administration of meloxicam 7.5 (A) or 15 (B) mg/day and comparison with IC_{50} values for COX-1 and COX-2. IC_{50} values for COX-1 and COX-2 inhibition in vitro were taken from Ref. 37, pharmacokinetic simulations were based on data from Ref. 42

was reduced by ~50%. However, none of these parameters were affected by meloxicam, 7.5 mg/day, confirming the COX-1 sparing effect in vivo in humans which was suggested by the simulations shown in Figures 1 and 2. Results with meloxicam, 15 mg/day, in similar experimental conditions are not yet available.

The differential inhibition of COX-1 and COX-2 by 100 mg nimesulide has been investigated in an ex vivo whole blood assay[37]. A maximal inhibition of COX-2(LPS-stimulated monocytes), accompanied by an ~50% inhibition of COX-1 (platelet TXB_2 synthesis) was observed, confirming previous clinical experience[46] and is also in agreement with the simulation shown in Figure 3. However, a subsequent study concluded that there was no significant effect of 100 mg nimesulide on serum TxB_2[47]. This discrepancy may be explained by the time points at which sampling was performed. In fact, due to the steep plasma concentration curve (Figure 3), very different results

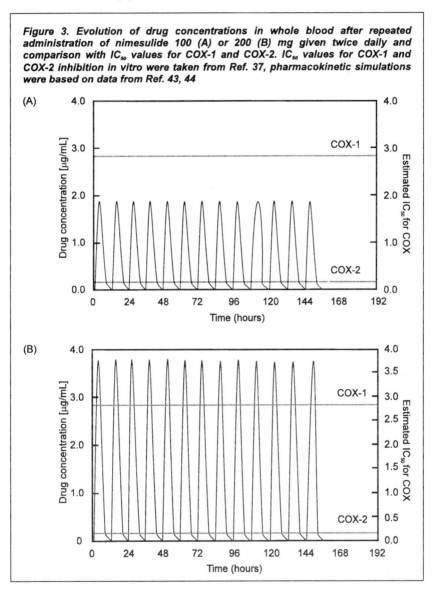

Figure 3. *Evolution of drug concentrations in whole blood after repeated administration of nimesulide 100 (A) or 200 (B) mg given twice daily and comparison with IC_{50} values for COX-1 and COX-2. IC_{50} values for COX-1 and COX-2 inhibition in vitro were taken from Ref. 37, pharmacokinetic simulations were based on data from Ref. 43, 44*

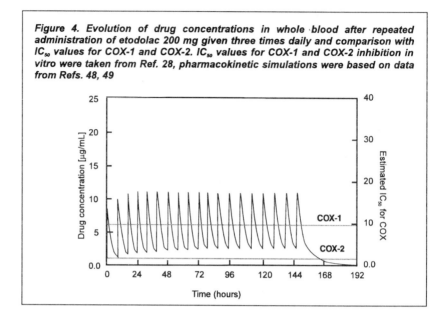

Figure 4. Evolution of drug concentrations in whole blood after repeated administration of etodolac 200 mg given three times daily and comparison with IC_{50} values for COX-1 and COX-2. IC_{50} values for COX-1 and COX-2 inhibition in vitro were taken from Ref. 28, pharmacokinetic simulations were based on data from Refs. 48, 49

may be obtained depending on the time point of sampling after drug administration. A similar observation is also applicable for etodolac, which is also characterized by a steep plasma concentration curve (Figure 4). In fact, studies performed with several non-selective 'standard' NSAIDs concluded that there was a close inverse relationship between plasma drug concentrations and serum TXB_2[50-55].

The selective COX-2 inhibitor MK 966, currently in clinical development, has also been tested in an ex vivo whole blood assay and no inhibition of COX-1 was shown at doses which blocked COX-2 activity completely[56].

The most relevant markers of COX-1 and COX-2 activity in vivo would be PGE_2 or PGI_2 production by the gastric mucosa and PGE_2 production by inflamed synovial tissue, respectively. However, practically, such studies are difficult to perform. These target tissues are not always easily obtainable and the methods used are prone to experimental error, since prostaglandin production occurs during tissue removal (when gastric mucosal or synovial biopsies are used). Furthermore, prostaglandin concentration in gastric juice or synovial fluid may not reflect precisely the synthetic activity of the gastric mucosa and synovial tissue, respectively. Nevertheless, early results suggest promising potential for a broad utilization of such methods[54,57-60], after an initial phase of validation and standardization.

CONCLUSIONS

From the results obtained using several in vitro test systems, NSAIDs can be classified as either non-selective compounds, which include the vast majority of standard NSAIDs currently used therapeutically, preferential inhibitors of COX-2, such as meloxicam, nimesulide and etodolac, or selective COX-2 inhibitors, including several pharmacological tools or developmental compounds such as flosulide, DuP-697, NS-398, L-745,337 and SC 58125. These conclusions are in agreement with the proposal for a new classification of NSAIDs according to their COX-2 selectivity rather than the usual chemical classification[61]. According to the results available, selective inhibition of COX-2 in vitro may translate into a COX-1 sparing effect at anti-inflammatory doses in vivo in humans. This also seems true for compounds with relative COX-2 selectivity (preferential inhibitors of COX-2), provided the plasma concentration curve is flat enough so that steady state levels are continuously maintained above the effective inhibitory concentrations for COX-2, but below the effective inhibitory concentrations for COX-1.

The in vitro and in vivo models commonly used to investigate the differential inhibition of COX-1 and COX-2 utilize platelets for COX-1 activity and stimulated monocytes for COX-2 activity. Future developments will include the use of cells or tissues closer to the target organs to investigate both therapeutic and side-effects in the clinic, such as gastric and synovial tissues, studied both in vitro and in vivo.

It is important to underline that in addition to COX-2 inhibition, NSAIDs may have other actions that contribute to their therapeutic effects[62,63]. Furthermore, mechanisms in addition to COX-1 inhibition, may also participate in the side-effects of these drugs[64,65]. It is therefore important to analyze the therapeutic relevance of selective COX-2 inhibition using large-scale head-to-head comparisons. Data on COX-2 selectivity can only provide a possible explanation for an improved gastro-intestinal tolerability but will not replace results from large scale clinical trials.

References

1. Fu JY, Masferrer JL, Seibert K, Raz A, Needleman P. The induction and suppression of prostaglandin H_2 synthase (cyclooxygenase) in human monocytes. J Biol Chem. 1990; 265: 16737–40.
2. Xie W, Chipman JG, Robertson DL, Erikson RL, Simmons DL. Expression of a mitogen-responsive gene encoding prostaglandin synthase is regulated by mRNA splicing. Proc Natl Acad Sci USA. 1991; 88: 1692–6.
3. Vane JR. Towards a better aspirin. Nature. 1994; 367: 215–16.
4. Pairet M, Engelhardt G. Distinct isoforms (COX-1 and COX-2) of cyclooxygenase: possible physiological and therapeutic implications. Fund Clin Pharmacol. 1996; 10: 1–15.
5. Euler US v. Zur Kenntnis der pharmakologischen Wirkungen von Nativsekreten und Extrakten männlicher accessorischer Geschlechtsdrüsen. Arch Exp Path Pharmakol. 1934; 975: 78–84.
6. Goldblatt MW. Properties of human seminal plasma. J Physiol (Lond). 1935; 84: 208–18.
7. Raz A, Wyche A, Siegel N, Needleman P. Regulation of fibroblast cyclooxygenase synthesis by interleukin-1. J Biol Chem. 1988; 263: 3022–5.
8. Sirois J, Levy LO, Simmons DL, Richards JS. Characterization and hormonal regulation of the promoter of the rat prostaglandin endoperoxide synthase 2 gene in granulosa cells. J Biol Chem. 1993; 268: 7384–5.
9. Slater D, Berger L, Newton R, Moore G, Bennett P. The relative abundance of type 1 to type 2 cyclo-oxygenase mRNA in human amnion at term. Biochem Biophys Res Commun. 1994; 198: 304–8.
10. Futaki N, Takahashi S, Yokoyama M, Arai I, Higuchi S, Otomo S. NS-398, a new anti-inflammatory agent, selectively inhibits prostaglandin G/H synthase/cyclooxygenase (COX-2) activity in vitro. Prostaglandins. 1994; 47: 55–9.

11. Ogino K, Harada Y, Kawamura M et al. An inhibitory effect of meloxicam, a novel non-steroidal anti-inflammatory drug, on COX-2. Jpn J Pharmacol. 1996; 71 (Suppl. 1): 304P.

12. Vago T, Bevilacqua M, Norbiato G. Effect of nimesulide action time dependence on selectivity towards prostaglandin G/H synthase/cyclooxygenase activity. Arzneim Forsch/Drug Res. 1995; 45: 1096–8.

13. Carbaza A, Cabré F, Rotllan E et al. Effect of COX-2 inhibitors on constitutive and inducible cyclooxygenase activity from different sources. Comparison with antiinflammatory activity. Prostaglandins, Leukotrienes Essential Fatty Acids. 1996; 55 (Suppl. 1): P93.

14. Klein T, Nüsing RM, Wiesenberg-Boettcher I, Ullrich V. Mechanistic studies on the selective inhibition of cyclooxygenase-2 by indanone derivatives. Biochem Pharmacol. 1996; 51: 285–90.

15. Mitchell JA, Akarasereenont P, Thiemermann C, Flower RJ, Vane JR. Selectivity of nonsteroidal antiinflammatory drugs as inhibitors of constitutive and inducible cyclooxygenase. Proc Natl Acad Sci USA. 1994; 90: 11693–7.

16. Pairet M, Lidbury PS, Engelhardt G, Trummlitz G, Vane JR. Meloxicam: cyclooxygenase selectivity, anti-inflammatory activity and gastric and renal safety. Inflamm Res. 1995; 44 (Suppl. 3): S274.

17. Klein T, Nüsing RM, Pfeilschifter J, Ullrich V. Selective inhibition of cyclooxygenase 2. Biochem Pharmacol. 1994; 48: 1605–10.

18. Engelhardt G, Bögel R, Schnitzler C, Utzman R. Meloxicam: influence on arachidonic acid metabolism: Part 1. In vitro findings. Biochem Pharmacol. 1996; 51: 21–8.

19. Meade EA, Smith WL, DeWitt DL. Differential inhibition of prostaglandin endoperoxide synthase (cyclooxygenase) isozymes by aspirin and other non-steroidal anti-inflammatory drugs. J Biol Chem. 1993; 268: 6610–14.

20. Seibert K, Zhang Y, Leahy K et al. Pharmacological and biochemical demonstration of the role of cyclooxygenase 2 in inflammation and pain. Proc Natl Acad Sci USA. 1994; 91: 12013–17.

21. Huff R, Collins P, Kramer S et al. A structural feature of N-[2–8cyclohexyloxy)-4-nitrophenyl] methanesulfonamide (NS-398) that governs its selectivity and affinity for cyclooxygenase 2(COX2). Inflamm Res. 1995; 44 (Suppl.2): S145–6.

22. Prasit P, Black WC, Chan CC et al. L-745,337: A selective cyclooxygenase-2 inhibitor. Med Chem Res. 1995; 5: 364–74.

23. Christoph T, Bodenteich A, Berg J. A whole cell assay system to test for specific COX inhibitors using the human monocytic cell line Mono Mac 6 and the human megacaryocytic cell line DAMI. Prostaglandins, Leukotrienes Essential Fatty Acids. 1996; 55 (Suppl.1): P3.

24. Barnett J, Chow J, Ives D et al. Purification, characterization and selective inhibition of human prostaglandin G/H synthase 1 and 2 expressed in the baculovirus system. Biochim Biophys Acta. 1994; 1209: 130–9.

25. Copeland RA, Williams JM, Giannaras J et al. Mechanism of selective inhibition of the inducible form of prostaglandin G/H synthase. Proc Natl Acad Sci USA. 1994; 91: 11202–6.

26. Laneuville O, Breuer DK, Dewitt DL, Hla T, Funk CD, Smith WD. Differential inhibition of human prostaglandin endoperoxide H synthases-1 and -2 by nonsteroidal anti-inflammatory drugs. J Pharmacol Exp Ther. 1994; 271: 927–34.

27. O'Neill GP, Mancini JA, Kargman S et al. Overexpression of human prostaglandin G/H synthase-1 and -2 by recombinant vaccinia virus: inhibition by nonsteroidal anti-inflammatory drugs and biosynthesis of 15-hydroxyeicosatetraenoic acid. Mol Pharmacol. 1994; 45: 245–54.

28. Glaser K, Sung ML, O'Neill K et al. Etodolac selectively inhibits human prostaglandin G/H synthase 2 (PGHS-2) versus human PGHS-1. Eur J Pharmacol. 1995; 281: 107–11.

29. Gierse JK, Hauser SD, Creely DP et al. Expression and selective inhibition of the constitutive and inducible forms of human cyclo-oxygenase. Biochem J. 1995; 305: 479–84.

30. Churchill L, Graham AG, Shih CK, Pauletti D, Farina PR, Grob PM. Selective inhibition of human cyclo-oxygenase-2 by meloxicam. Inflammopharmacol. 1996; 4: 125–35.

31. Cromlish WA, Kennedy BP. Selective inhibition of cyclooxygenase-1 and -2 using intact insect cell assays. Biochem Pharmacol. 1996; 52: 1777–85.

32. Kargman S, Wong E, Greig GM et al. Mechanism of selective inhibition of human prostaglandin G/H synthase-1 and -2 in intact cells. Biochem Pharmacol. 1996; 52: 1113–25.

33. Tavares IA, Bennett A. Acemetacin and indomethacin: Differential inhibition of constitutive and inducible cyclo-oxygenases in human gastric mucosa and leucocytes. Int J Tiss Reac. 1993; 15: 49–53.
34. Tavares IA, Bishai PM, Bennett A. Activity of nimesulide on constitutive and inducible cyclooxygenases. Arzneim Forsch/Drug Res. 1995; 45: 1093–5.
35. Grossman CJ, Wiseman J, Lucas FS, Trevethick MA, Birch PJ. Inhibition of constitutive and inducible cyclooxygenase activity in human platelets and mononuclear cells by NSAIDs and Cox 2 inhibitors. Inflamm Res. 1995; 44: 253–7.
36. Patrignani P, Panara MR, Greco A et al. Biochemical and pharmacological characterization of the cyclooxygenase activity of human blood prostaglandin endoperoxide synthases. J Pharmacol Exp Ther. 1994; 271: 1705–10.
37. Patrignani P, Panara MR, Santini G et al. Differential inhibition of cyclooxygenase activity of prostaglandin endoperoxide synthase isozymes *in vitro* and *ex vivo* in man. Prostaglandins, Leukotrienes Essential Fatty Acids. 1996; 55 (Suppl.1): P115.
38. Young JM, Panah S, Satchawatcharaphong C, Cheung PS. Human whole blood assays for inhibition of prostaglandin G/H synthases-1 and -2 using A23187 and lipopolysaccharide stimulation of thromboxane B2 production. Inflamm Res. 1996; 45: 246–53.
39. Brideau C, Kargman S, Liu S et al. A human whole blood assay for clinical evaluation of biochemical efficacy of cyclooxygenase inhibitors. Inflamm Res. 1996; 45: 68–74.
40. Hayllar J, Bjarnason I. NSAIDs, Cox-2 inhibitors, and the gut. Lancet 1995; 346: 521–2.
41. Rabasseda X. Nimesulide: a selective cyclooxygenase 2 inhibitor antiinflammatory drug. Drugs of Today. 1996; 32 (Suppl.D): 1–23.
42. Türck D, Bursch U, Heinzel G, Narjes HH. Clinical pharmacokinetics of meloxicam. Arzneim Forsch/Drug Res. 1997; 47: 253–8.
43. Theiss U, Timmer W, Wieckhorst G, Macciocchi A, Wetzelsberger N. Investigation into a possible drug–drug interaction between warfarin and nimesulide in healthy volunteers. Methods Find Exp Clin Pharmacol. 1993; 15: 629–35.
44. Davis R, Brodgen RN. Nimesulide. An update of its pharmacodynamic and pharmacokinetic properties, and therapeutic efficacy. Drugs. 1994; 48: 431–54.
45. Stichtenoth DO, Wagner B, Frölich JC. Effects of meloxicam and indomethacin on cyclooxygenase pathways in healthy volunteers. J Invest Med. 1997; in press.
46. Ward A, Brogden RN. Nimesulide: A preliminary review of its pharmacological properties and therapeutic efficacy in inflammation and pain states. Drugs. 1988; 36: 732–5.
47. Cullen L, Kelly L, Coyle D, Forde R, Fitzgerald D. Selective suppression of COX-2 during chronic administration of nimesulide in man. William Harvey Research Conference: Selective COX-2 inhibitors: Pharmacology, clinical effects and therapeutic potential, Cannes 20th-21st March 1997; Abstract.
48. Brater DC. Profile of Etodolac: Pharmacokinetic evaluation in special populations. Clin Rheumatol. 1989; 8 (Suppl.1): 25–35.
49. Brocks DR, Jamali F. Etodolac Clinical Pharmacokinetics. Clin Pharmacokinet. 1994; 26: 259–74.
50. Rane A, Oelz O, Frölich JC et al. Relationship between plasma concentrations of indomethacin and its effect on prostaglandin synthesis and platelet aggregation in man. Clin Pharmacol Ther. 1978; 23: 658–68.
51. Cronberg S, Wallmark E, Södeberg I. Effect on platelet aggregation of oral administration of 10 non-steroidal analgesics to humans. Scand J Haematol. 1984; 33: 155–9.
52. Vinge E. Arachidonic acid-induced platelet aggregation and prostanoid formation in whole blood in relation to plasma concentration of indomethacin. Eur J Clin Pharmacol. 1985; 28: 163–9.
53. Cox SR, Vanderlugt JT, Gumbleton TJ, Smith RB. Relationships between thromboxane production, platelet aggregability, and serum concentrations of ibuprofen and flurbiprofen. Clin Pharmacol Ther. 1987; 41: 510–21.
54. Day RO, Francis H, Vial J, Geisslinger G, Williams KM. Naproxen concentrations in plasma and synovial fluid and effects on prostanoid concentrations. J Rheumatol. 1995; 22: 2295–303.
55. Schafer AI. Effects of nonsteroidal antiinflammatory drugs on platelet function and systemic hemostasis. J Clin Pharmacol. 1995; 35: 209–19.

56. Ehrich E, Dallob A, Van Hecken A et al. Demonstration of selective COX-2 inhibition by MK-966 in humans. Arthritis Rheum. 1996; 39 (Suppl.): Abstract 328.
57. Faust TW, Redfern JS, Podolsky I, Lee E, Grundy SM, Feldman M. Effects of aspirin on gastric mucosal prostaglandin E_2 and $F_{2\alpha}$ content and on gastric mucosal injury in humans receiving fish oil or olive oil. Gastroenterology. 1990; 98: 586–91.
58. Taha AS, McLaughlin S, Holland PJ, Kelly RW, Sturrock RD, Russell RI. Effect on gastric and duodenal mucosal prostaglandins of repeated intake of therapeutic doses of naproxen and etodolac in rheumatoid arthritis. Ann Rheum Dis. 1990; 49: 354–8.
59. Hudson N, Balsitis M, Filipowicz F, Hawkey C. Effect of *Helicobacter pylori* colonisation on gastric mucosal eicosanoid synthesis in patients taking non-steroidal anti-inflammatory drugs. Gut. 1993; 34: 748–51.
60. Bertin P, Lapicque F, Payan E et al. Sodium naproxen: concentration and effect on inflammatory response mediators in human rheumatoid synovial fluid. Clin Pharmacol. 1994; 46: 3–7.
61. Frölich JC. A classification of NSAIDs according to the relative inhibition of cyclooxygenase isoenzymes. Trends in Pharmacol Sci. 1997; 18: 30–4.
62. Brooks PM, Day RO. Nonsteroidal antiinflammatory drugs – differences and similarities. N Engl J Med. 1991; 324: 1716–25.
63. Insel P. Analgesic-antipyretic and antiinflammatory agents and drugs employed in the treatment of gout. In: Hardman JG, Limbird LE, Molinoff PB, Ruddon RW, Goodman Gilman A (eds). Goodman & Gilman's Pharmacological Basis of Therapeutics. 9th edn; 1995: 617–57.
64. Lichtenstein D, Syngal S, Wolfe MM. Nonsteroidal antiinflammatory drugs and the gastrointestinal tract. Arthritis Rheum. 1995; 38: 5–18.
65. Mahmud T, Scott DL, Bjarnason I. A unifying hypothesis for the mechanism of NSAID related gastrointestinal toxicity. Ann Rheum Dis. 1996; 55: 211–13.

4 COX-2 in brain and retina: role in neuronal survival

N.G. BAZAN, V.L. MARCHESELLI, P.K. MUKHERJEE, W.J. LUKIW, W.C. GORDON and D. ZHANG

Various forms of injury to the central nervous system, such as in neurodegenerative diseases, sets in motion an inflammatory-like response. The messengers that accumulate are normal modulators of functions; however, above certain concentrations they trigger neuronal damage. The significance of these early warning events has recently been highlighted by the observation that patients receiving chronic treatments with certain anti-inflammatory drugs develop less severe symptoms of Alzheimer's Disease. Cyclooxygenase-2 (COX-2) and platelet-activating factor (PAF), mediators of the inflammatory response, may thus play a role in Alzheimer's Disease and in other neurodegenerative diseases.

PAF (1–0-alkyl-sn-2-acetyl-3-phosphocholine), the most potent biologically active lipid known, is involved in the injury/inflammatory response in many cells. In brain, PAF is rapidly produced at the onset of ischaemia and seizures. PAF, the only bioactive phospholipid to have a cloned receptor, also elicits actions through an intracellular site. Physiologically, PAF modulates glutamate release, long-term potentiation (LTP) and memory formation. Furthermore, PAF is a transcriptional activator of COX-2. Interestingly, COX-2 as well as PAF, is involved in both synaptic plasticity (e.g. LTP) and in the injury/inflammatory response. Unlike in other cells, however, COX-2 is constitutively expressed in neurons at low levels.

Two CNS disease rat models were investigated to determine whether COX-2 is induced under pathological conditions and whether the antagonist that blocks PAF-induction of the COX-2 promoter inhibits kainic acid-induced epileptogenesis in vivo. There was sustained upregulation of COX-2 in the hippocampus, several-fold greater than another early response gene, *zif*-268. Pretreatment of animals with the intracellular PAF antagonist BN 50730 strongly attenuates COX-2 induction. In the second model, light-induced photoreceptor cell COX-2 protein accumulates, preceding apoptotic nuclear changes, and localizes to inner segments of photoreceptor cells. The PAF antagonist significantly reduces COX-2 light induction and apoptosis. Currently, we are testing the hypothesis that the overexpression of the PAF-COX-2 pathway leads to neuronal cell apoptosis.

Although it is often stated that the inflammatory response is not associated with apoptotic cell death, PAF and COX-2 appear to act as neuronal injury messengers without inducing classical 'inflammatory' features in the entire tissue.

PLATELET ACTIVATING FACTOR AND OTHER BIOACTIVE LIPIDS

An important target for cerebral ischaemia (as in stroke and neurotrauma) and seizures (as in epilepsy) is phospholipids from plasma membranes of neural cells. Phospholipid molecules of membranes from neurons and glial cells store a wide variety of lipid messengers. Receptor-mediated events and changes in intracellular [Ca^{2+}], such as those occurring during excitatory neurotransmission and activity-dependent synaptic plasticity, activate phospholipases that catalyse the release of bioactive moieties from phospholipids. These messengers then participate in intracellular and/or intercellular signalling pathways. Bioactive lipids have significant neurobiological actions in neurotransmitter release, synaptic plasticity, and programmes of neuronal gene expression. Accordingly, contemporary research into bioactive lipids has focused on their neurobiological significance.

Cerebral ischaemia or seizure disrupts the tightly regulated events that control the production and accumulation of lipid messengers, such as free arachidonic acid, diacylglycerol and PAF, under physiological conditions (Figure 1). Rapid activation of phospholipases, particularly of phospholipase A$_2$ (PLA$_2$), occurs at the onset of cerebral ischaemia or seizures involved during these pathophysiological conditions[1]. There is a wide variety of PLA$_2$s[2], and current investigations aim to define those affected by ischaemia. For example, in addition to the role(s) of intracellular PLA$_2$s in lipid messenger formation, it has recently been discovered that a low molecular weight secretory PLA$_2$ increases glutamate-induced neuronal damage[3]. Whereas

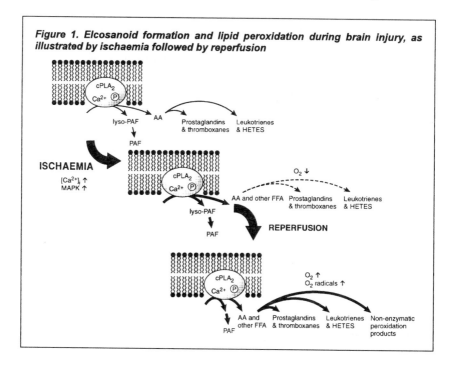

Figure 1. Eicosanoid formation and lipid peroxidation during brain injury, as illustrated by ischaemia followed by reperfusion

pathways leading to PLA_2 activation and release are part of normal neuronal function, ischaemia–reperfusion enhances these events, resulting in overproduction of PLA_2-derived lipid messengers (e.g. enzymatically produced arachidonic acid oxygenation metabolites, nonenzymatically generated lipid peroxidation products and other reactive oxygen species), involved in neuronal damage. Among the consequences of PLA_2 activation by ischaemia are alterations in mitochondrial function by the rapid increase in the brain free fatty acid pool size (e.g. uncoupling of oxidative phosphorylation from respiratory chain) and the generation of lipid messengers.

PAF is a very potent and short-lived lipid messenger which has a wide range of actions: as a mediator of inflammatory and immune responses, as a second messenger, and as a potent inducer of gene expression in neural systems. Thus, in addition to its acute roles, PAF can potentially mediate longer-term effects on cellular physiology and brain functions. In this chapter the significance of PAF in synaptic function and neuronal gene expression as they relate to cerebral ischaemia are discussed.

PAF MODULATES GLUTAMATE RELEASE AND SYNAPTIC PLASTICITY

PAF enhances glutamate release in synaptically paired rat hippocampal neurons in culture[4]. The PAF analogue methylcarbamyl-PAF (mc-PAF), but not biologically inactive lyso-PAF, increases excitatory synaptic responses. The inhibitory neurotransmitter γ-aminobutyric acid is unaffected by mc-PAF under these conditions. The presynaptic PAF receptor antagonist BN 52021 blocks the mc-PAF-enhanced glutamate release. In addition, mc-PAF increases presynaptic glutamate release, since it does not augment the effects of exogenously added glutamate, and it evokes spontaneous synaptic responses characteristic of enhanced neurotransmitter release. Therefore, as a modulator of glutamate release, PAF participates in long-term potentiation[5], synaptic plasticity and memory formation.

PAF contributes to excitotoxicity by enhancing glutamate release

Ischaemia and seizures increase PAF levels in brain[1]. Furthermore, the brain is endowed with a variety of degradative enzymes that rapidly convert PAF to biologically inactive lyso-PAF[6]. Presynaptic membranes display PAF binding that can be displaced by BN 52021, a terpenoid extracted from the leaf of the *Ginkgo biloba* tree which binds preferentially to the synaptosomal site[7]. It is likely that this PAF binding site is the seven-transmembrane PAF receptor that has been cloned by T. Shimizu et al.[1]. BN 52021 inhibits both PAF-induced glutamate release[4] and long-term potentiation[5]. Moreover, this antagonist is neuroprotective against ischaemia–reperfusion damage in the gerbil brain[1]. Taking these findings together, PAF, when overproduced at the synapse during ischaemia, will promote enhanced glutamate release that in turn, through the activation of postsynaptic receptors, will contribute to excitotoxicity.

PAF IS A TRANSCRIPTIONAL ACTIVATOR OF COX-2

In addition to its modulatory effect on synaptic transmission and neural plasticity, PAF activates receptor-mediated immediate early gene expression. Since PAF is a phospholipid and can pass through membranes, it is rapidly taken up by cells. An intracellular binding site with very high affinity, yet pharmacologically distinct from the presynaptic site, was found in brain[7]. The synthetic hetrazepine BN 50730 is selective for this intracellular site and blocks PAF-induced gene expression of the inducible COX-2 in transfected cells[8].

COX-2 catalyses the cyclooxygenation and peroxidation of arachidonic acid into PGH_2 the precursor of biologically active PGs, thromboxanes and prostacyclin. COX-1 also catalyses the same first committed step of the arachidonic acid cascade. COX-2, however, is expressed in response to mitogenic and inflammatory stimuli and is encoded by an early response gene. In contrast, COX-1 expression is not subject to short-term regulation. Neurones in the hippocampus, as well as in a few other brain regions, are unlike other cells in that they display basal levels of COX-2 expression[9]. This expression is modulated by synaptic activity, LTP and involves the N-methyl-D-aspartate class of glutamate receptors[9,10](Figure 2).

PAF is a transcriptional activator of COX-2, as PAF induces mouse COX-2 promoter-driven luciferase activity transfected in neuroblastoma cells (NG108–15 or SH-SY5Y) and in NIH 3T3 cells. The intracellular PAF antagonist, BN 50730, inhibits PAF activation of this construct[8].

SUSTAINED TRANSCRIPTIONAL UPREGULATION OF PGS-2 PRECEDES KAINIC ACID-INDUCED NEURONAL DAMAGE IN HIPPOCAMPUS

The abundant early-response gene transcripts in brain show rapid and transient increases during cerebral ischaemia and after seizures. Several early-response genes

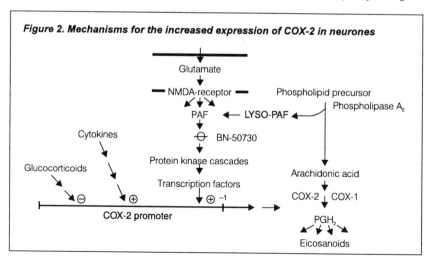

Figure 2. Mechanisms for the increased expression of COX-2 in neurones

encode transcription factors which in turn modulate the expression of other genes, whereas others encode inducible enzymes. The glutamate analogue kainic acid promotes extensive neuronal damage, particularly in the hippocampus, and also induces early-response genes such as the transcription factor *zif*-268. COX-2 is also induced under these conditions, but there are striking differences in the magnitude and duration of the induction of COX-2 as compared with *zif*-268. Two hours after kainic acid injection COX-2 mRNA showed a 35-fold increase in hippocampus, compared with only a 5.5-fold increase in *zif*-268[11]. The peak in COX-2 mRNA was evident at 3 hours (71-fold increase), compared with 1 hour for *zif*-268 (10-fold increase). The time-course of *zif*-268 mRNA changes in the hippocampus corresponds to the expected profile of early-response genes, i.e. a rapid decrease in abundance after the peak. COX-2, on the other hand, displayed sustained up-regulation for several hours after kainic acid injection (5.2-fold increase at 12 hours)[11].

THE PLATELET ACTIVATING FACTOR-PROSTAGLANDIN G/H SYNTHASE-2 INTRACELLULAR SIGNALLING PATHWAY AND POSSIBLE COX-2 SUBTYPES

A PAF-stimulated signal transduction pathway is a major component of kainic acid-induced COX-2 expression in hippocampus. This conclusion is based upon the findings that PAF induces mouse COX-2 promoter-driven luciferase activity in transfected cells, and BN 50730 inhibits this effect[8] and that BN 50730 (given intracerebroventricularly 15 minutes before kainic acid) inhibits kainic acid-induced COX-2 mRNA accumulation in hippocampus by 90%[8]. Both PAF[12] and COX-2[13] are potent mediators of the injury/inflammatory response. PAF[4,5] and COX-2[9,10] are also interrelated in neuronal plasticity. The sequence of events that leads to synaptic activation of COX-2 may be initiated by NMDA-ionotropic glutamate receptor activation followed by PAF production. The bioactive lipid will, through protein kinase cascades[14] and transcription factors[15], promote the transcriptional activation of COX-2. NMDA-activated COX-2 and its linkage to synaptic plasticity has been suggested[9,10]. It is of interest that this COX-2 species seems to be related to function, as is PAF, in long-term potentiation[4,5] and memory[16,17]. This physiological COX-2 seems to be located in dendrites, whereas another COX-2 species seems to be located in the perinuclear region of neurones[10]. Subtypes of COX-2, or perhaps a COX-3, may be present in neurones, one being a physiological gene product linked to LTP and function (dendritic) and the other a COX that greatly increases as a result of pathological stimulation (perinuclear). Transcriptional regulatory mechanisms, as well as COX-2 structural/localization signals, may underlie these differences. The pathological COX-2 species may be represented by the protein overexpressed in injury situations such as during kainic acid-induced status epilepticus. Although COX-2 is an early response gene and this class of genes is known to be increased during seizures[18–22], COX-2 exhibits a 72-fold increase after kainic acid in vivo in the hippocampus[11] compared with a 10-fold increase in *zif*-268, a gene encoding a zinc finger containing transcription factor. There is, therefore, something unique in the COX-2 gene transcriptional controlling events which are so sensitive to pathological stimulation. Ischaemia–reperfusion exerts a similar action[22], indicating a role for COX-2 in stroke. Major therapeutic issues emerge from these studies concerning the use of selective COX-2 inhibitors for many systemic inflammatory diseases. First of all, will these drugs, by crossing the blood–brain barrier, affect the physiological COX-2? Second, an inflammatory component where COX-2 may play a role has been hypothesized in neurodegenerative diseases such as Alzheimer's[23]. Therefore, selective COX-2 inhibitors may become useful. However, once the overproduction of brain COX-2 is set in motion, will selective COX-2 inhibitors be of help? Would it be better to design drugs that block the pathological transcriptional up-regulation of brain COX-2? This alternative may also have the merit of not interfering with the physiological COX-2 species. The PAF transcriptional activation of COX-2 may also provide novel clues about neuronal cell death pathways. The antagonist BN 50730 was much less effective against *zif*-268 expression. In fact, the delayed hippocampal induction of COX-2 by kainic acid precedes selective neuronal apoptosis by this agonist in this neuroanatomical region.

In cerebrovascular diseases the significance of the PLA_2-related signalling triggered by ischaemia–reperfusion may be part of events finely balanced between neuroprotection and neuronal cell death. The precise events that would tilt this balance toward the latter are currently being explored. It is interesting to note that PAF, being short-lived and rapidly degraded by PAF acetylhydrolase[6], is a long-term signal with consequences for neurones through sustained COX-2 expression. COX-2 is localized in the nuclear envelope and perinuclear endoplasmic reticulum. The overexpression of hippocampal COX-2 during cerebral ischaemia and seizures may in turn lead to the formation of neurotoxic metabolites (e.g. superoxide). Current investigations aim to determine whether or not other messengers cooperate to enhance neuronal damage (e.g. nitric oxide) and the possible involvement of astrocytes and microglial cells. Further understanding of these potentially neurotoxic events involving lipid messengers and COX-2 will permit the identification of new strategies and define therapeutic windows for the management of cerebrovascular and neurodegenerative diseases.

Acknowledgements

This work was supported by NIH grant NS23002.

References

1. Bazan NG, Rodriguez de Turco EB, Allan G. Mediators of injury in neurotrauma: Intracellular signal transduction and gene expression. J Neurotrauma. 1995; 12: 789–911.
2. Dennis EA. Diversity of group types, regulation and function of phospholipase A_2. J Biol Chem. 1994; 269: 13057–60.
3. Kolko M, DeCoster MA, Rodriguez de Turco EB. Synergy by secretory phospholipase A_2 and glutamate on inducing cell death and sustained arachidonic acid metabolic changes in primary cortical neuronal cultures. J Biol Chem. 1996; 271: 32722–8.
4. Clark GD, Happel LT, Zorumski CF, Bazan NG. Enhancement of hippocampal excitatory synaptic transmission by platelet-activating factor. Neuron. 1992; 9: 1211–16.

5. Kaufmann WE, Worley PF, Pegg J, Bremer M, Isakson P. COX-2, a synaptically induced enzyme, is expressed by excitatory neurons at postsynaptic sites in rat cerebral cortex. Proc Natl Acad Sci USA. 1996; 93: 2317–21.

6. Bazan NG. Inflammation: A signal terminator. Nature. 1995; 374: 501–2.

7. Marcheselli VL, Rossowska M, Domingo MT, Braquet P, Bazan NG. Distinct platelet-activating factor binding sites in synaptic endings and in intracellular membranes of rat cerebral cortex. J Biol Chem. 1990; 265: 9140–5.

8. Bazan NG, Fletcher BS, Herschman HR, Mukherjee PK. Platelet-activating factor and retinoic acid synergistically activate the inducible prostaglandin synthase gene. Proc Natl Acad Sci USA. 1994; 91: 5252–6.

9. Yamagata K, Andreasson KI, Kaufmann WE, Barnes CA, Worley PF. Expression of a mitogen-inducible cyclooxygenase in brain neurons: Regulation by synaptic activity and glucocorticoids. Neuron. 1993; 11: 371–86.

10. Kato K, Clark GD, Bazan NG, Zorumski CF. Platelet activating factor as a potential retrograde messenger in Ca^1 hippocampal long-term potentiation. Nature. 1994; 367: 175–9.

11. Marcheselli VL, Bazan NG. Sustained induction of prostaglandin endoperoxide synthase-2 by seizures in hippocampus. Inhibition by a platelet-activating factor antagonist. J Biol Chem. 1996; 271: 24794–9.

12. Prescott SM, Zimmerman GA, McIntyre TM. Platelet-activating factor. J Biol Chem. 1990; 265: 17381–4.

13. Bazan NG, Botting J, Vane JR (Eds.) New Targets in Inflammation: Inhibitors of COX-2 or Adhesion Molecules. London: William Harvey Press, and Lancaster: Kluwer Academic Publishers, 1996.

14. Mukherjee PK, DeCoster MA, Davis RJ, Bazan NG. Differential activation of p38, JNK, and mitogen-activated protein kinases (MAPKs) by platelet-activating factor (PAF), glutamate (GLU), and kainate (KA) in primary hippocampal neurons. Experimental Biology, New Orleans, LA, April 6–9, 1997.

15. Lukiw WJ, Gordon WC, Bazan NG. Levels of transcription factor AP1, AP2, SP1, GAS-, NFKB- and TFIID-DNA binding during rat retinal neovascularization. Invest Ophthalmol Vis Sci. 1997; 38 (Suppl.): S611.

16. Izquierdo I, Fin C, Schmitz PK et al. Memory enhancement by intrahippocampal, intraamygdala, or intraentorhinal infusion of platelet-activating factor measured in an inhibitory avoidance task. Proc Natl Acad Sci USA. 1995; 92: 5047–51.

17. Packard MG, Teather L, Bazan NG. Effects of intrastriatal injections of platelet-activating factor and the PAF antagonist BN 52021 on memory. Neurobiol Learn Mem. 1996; 66: 177–82.

18. Bazan NG, Doucet JP. Platelet-activating factor and intracellular signaling pathways that modulate gene expression. In: Shukla S, (ed.) Platelet-Activating Factor Receptors: Signal Mechanisms and Molecular Biology, Boca Raton, FL: CRC Press, 1993: 137–46.

19. Doucet JP, Bazan NG. A neural primary genomic response to the lipid mediator plateletactivating factor. In R Massarelli, LA Horrocks, JN Kanfer, R Loffelholz, (eds). Phospholipids and Signal Transmission vol 70. Berlin–Heidelberg, Springer Verlag. 1993: 411–26.

20. Doucet JP, Squinto SP, Bazan NG. FOX-JUN and the primary genomic response in the nervous system: Physiological role and pathophysiological significance. Mol Neurobiol. 1990; 4: 27–55.

21. Doucet JP, Bazan NG. Excitable membranes, lipid messengers, and immediate-early genes: Alteration of signal transduction in neuromodulation and neurotrauma. Mol Neurobiol. 1992; 6: 407–24.

22. Collaco-Moraes Y, Aspey B, Harrison M, de Belleroche J: Cyclo-oxygenase-2 messenger RNA induction in focal cerebral ischemia. J Cerebr Blood Flow Metab. 1996; 16: 1366–72.

23. Lukiw WJ, Bazan NG. Cyclooxygenase-2 (COX-2) RNA message stability in Alzheimer's Disease (AD) neocortex. Society for Neuroscience, New Orleans, LA, October 25–30, 1997.

5 COX-2 and apoptosis: NSAIDs as effectors of programmed cell death

D.L. SIMMONS, M.L. MADSEN and P.M. ROBERTSON

For decades it has been recognized that growth and development, as well as the maintenance of appropriate cell numbers in adult multicellular organisms, is dependent not only on proper cell division but also on a carefully regulated programme of cell death (apoptosis). Increasing evidence suggests that abnormal hyperproliferative diseases such as neoplasia result not only from aberrations in the inability of the cell to halt cell division, but also in cellular deficiencies in the processes leading to senescence and cell death.

Whether in tadpole tails experiencing resorption during metamorphosis or in the mitotically active colonic crypts of mammals, where epithelial cells proliferate and then die, apoptosis occurs through a highly evolutionarily conserved cascade of biochemical events. These events can be initiated by a wide variety of agents, including cell–cell interactions, hormones, cytokines and drugs. Initiators of apoptosis can be highly specific for certain cell types and may have no apoptotic effects in other cells. In contrast, these multiple signalling pathways funnel down to a conserved core signalling pathway controlling cell death. Ultimate cellular processes triggered by this pathway are scission of genomic DNA, crosslinking of cellular proteins, mitochondrial cell death, membrane blebbing and the formation of apoptotic bodies, the hallmarks of apoptosis[1].

CYCLOOXYGENASES AND APOPTOSIS

Prostaglandin (PG)H_2 generated by cyclooxygenases (COX)-1 and -2 is isomerized into common prostaglandins that have been found to be apoptotic in lymphocytes. PGE2, potently induces apoptosis in T and B cells[2,3] and is able to antagonize activation-induced apoptosis in T cells. Prostaglandins that are yet undefined are also involved in programmed cell death of epithelial cells of the basement membrane of the uterus during implantation and of ovarian epithelial cells that cover the surface of the preovulatory follicle[4,5]. The roles of COX-1 and COX-2 in these instances are to initiate synthesis of these PGs which presumably act as paracrine factors that instigate apoptosis signalling through their respective cell surface receptors. PGA_2 and Δ^{12}-PGJ_2 also cause apoptosis in lymphocytes but have no cell surface receptor and possibly act through intracellular sites such as the peroxisome proliferator-activated receptor(PPAR)-γ transcription factor[6,7].

INDUCTION OF APOPTOSIS BY NON-STEROID ANTI-INFLAMMATORY DRUGS

COXs do not regulate apoptosis solely as synthesizers of apoptosis-inducing prostaglandins in lymphoid cells. Non-steroid anti-inflammatory drugs (NSAIDs) that are competitive inhibitors of COX-1 and COX-2, and which completely inhibit PGG_2 and PGH_2 synthesis by occluding the cyclooxygenation site of these bifunctional enzymes, uniformly induce apoptosis in susceptible cells in culture. Rodent and human cell lines from neoplastic and normal colonic epithelial cells[8–13], v-*src* transformed chicken embryo fibroblasts[14] and murine macrophage cells (the J774 cell line, unpublished data) have been demonstrated to be sensitive to NSAID-induced apoptosis (NIA). The lung carcinoma cell line, A549, is resistant (unpublished data).

Aspirin, the prototypical NSAID, does not cause apoptosis except at very high doses (>1 mM) where it, or its metabolite salicylate, probably acts as a competitive COX inhibitor[11]. Typically, aspirin acts as a non-competitive COX inhibitor by acetylating Ser^{530} to partially block the cyclooxygenation site. The fact that partial blocking of the cyclooxygenation site by aspirin is insufficient to cause apoptosis, although it completely inhibits prostaglandin synthesis, suggests that inhibition of prostaglandins *per se* is not the mechanism by which NSAIDs cause NIA and that synthesis of the metabolite that mediates NIA is not blocked by aspirin acetylation. This latter point would indicate that the cyclooxygenation site of the acetylated COX enzyme is large enough to accommodate the substrate producing this putative mediator, suggesting either that this substrate is smaller than arachidonic acid or is only partially oxygenated, as is the case with 15-(R)-HETE, which is made by COX-2 that has been acetylated by aspirin treatment[15].

THE CELLULAR AND BIOCHEMICAL PHENOTYPE OF NIA

As with other forms of apoptosis, NIA exhibits sequential cellular and biochemical changes resulting in or accompanying cell death. In all cells thus far examined, DNA fragmentation to nucleosomal ladders is observed[8–14]. In v-*src*-transformed CEF this has been shown to be preceded by cleavage of the DNA to high molecular weight fragments. Another marked change is that the cells round and become less adherent to the substratum. Nuclear anomalies are evident and during the terminal stages of apoptosis extensive membrane blebbing and the formation of apoptotic bodies is evident[8–14].

Numerous biochemical events have been associated with cell death. Some of these molecular members of signal transduction pathways have been demonstrated to directly regulate NIA in a positive or negative fashion. Induction of c-*myc* is clearly required for NIA in CEF as shown by the fact that anti-sense oligonucleotide inhibition of c-*myc* expression prevents NIA. The oncogene v-*src* also potentiates NIA in these cells, as shown by the fact that a temperature-sensitive mutant of v-*src* greatly increases NIA at the permissive temperature (37°C). The proto-oncogene *bcl*-2 also directly regulates NIA in CEF that normally have very low levels of this protein. In this case, *bcl*-2 expression blocks NIA from occurring as shown by the fact that overexpression of human *bcl-2* using a retroviral expression vector completely prevents NIA[16].

NSAIDs THAT CAUSE NIA ALSO INDUCE COX-2 IN CEF AND MAMMALIAN CELLS

Among known alterations in gene expression occurring during NIA are some changes that are particularly intriguing with regard to the pharmacology of NSAIDs and the known anti-neoplastic effects of these drugs. One of these is the finding that competitively acting NSAIDs induce COX-2 mRNA and protein[14]. With the exception of diclofenac, these drugs do not induce COX-1 mRNA and protein and in some cases they decrease their levels. Concentrations of NSAIDs that have this inductive effect are physiologically relevant, and in CEF maximum induction is observed at concentrations near 25–50 µM. At increasing dose levels of NSAIDs striking alteration in splicing of the COX-2 pre-mRNA is seen (Figure 1). At NSAID doses >100 µM, COX-2 expression decreases and an increasing percentage of COX-2 mRNA is expressed as a non-functional splicing variant in which intron 1 is left unspliced[16]. As described later, intron 1 in chicken is distinctly different in its organization and sequence from intron 1 in mammalian COX-2 genes. However, the striking regulation

Figure 1. Effect of concentration on diclofenac induction of COX-1 and COX-2. *For Northern blot analysis, 20 µg of total RNA from RSV-transformed CEFs with and without treatment with various doses of diclofenac 29 hours after shift to 37°C, was hybridized to COX-1, COX-2, or GAPDH probes. Lanes: 1, serum-starved RSV-transformed cells without drug treatment; 2–6, diclofenac treatment at 25 µM, 50 µM, 100 µM, 200 µM, and 400 µM, respectively. COX-1, 7 day exposure; COX-2, 20 hours' exposure; GAPDH, 6 hours' exposure*

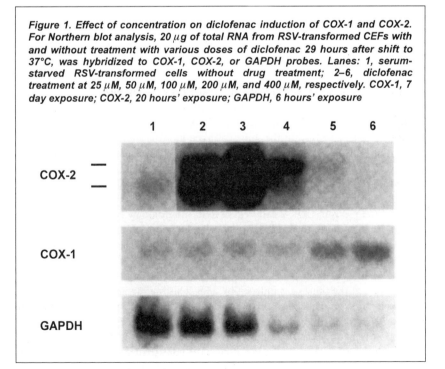

of splicing of this COX-2 intron further substantiates the selective role this isoenzyme plays in the apoptosis process.

Murine J774.2 cells but not NIA-refractory A549 cells also exhibit markedly elevated COX-2, but not COX-1 protein after chronic treatment with competitive NSAIDs. High doses of aspirin (2–4 mM) also weakly induce COX-2 protein in these cells but paracetamol has no effect.

CONCOMITANT WITH ELEVATION OF COX-2 mRNA AND PROTEIN IS AN INDUCTION OF A NOVEL COX-2 ACTIVITY

The marked increase in COX-2 mRNA and protein observed in CEF due to chronic treatment with competitively acting NSAIDs such as diclofenac was anticipated to be catalytically inactive. This supposition was based on the fact that relatively high concentrations of drug were used to induce NIA and because many of these drugs (e.g. diclofenac, indomethacin, flurbiprofen, etc.) are known to essentially irreversibly bind the cyclooxygenation site of purified COX, as well as COX found in non-apoptotic cells. To test for activity in cells undergoing NIA, J774.2 cells were treated for 48 hours with increasing doses of diclofenac, rapidly washed twice to remove the drug, and COX activity was then measured. In multiple replications of this experiment low concentrations of drug consistently inhibited COX activity, but high (apoptotic) concentrations increased it. When COX activity in the respective treatment groups was normalized for cell number, an enormous induction of cyclooxygenase activity was evident at NSAID concentrations above 250 µM. We also found a large increase in COX activity in v-src-transformed CEF treated with the same regimen.

This NSAID-induced COX activity in J774.2 cells is inhibited by the NSAID that induced it as well as by other non-aspirin NSAIDs. However, high concentrations of drug are needed to inhibit this induced COX activity than are required for inhibition of either COX-1 or COX-2 in the same cell type growing under normal conditions. Furthermore, this NIA-induced activity is completely insensitive to inhibition by aspirin. At present we have been unable to dissociate induction of COX-2 and the NSAID-induced COX activity, suggesting that they are either coordinately regulated or the same entity. However, all of our data suggest that NSAID-inducible COX is distinctly different from COX-2 with regard to its inhibition by NSAIDs. Therefore, if COX-2 is the NSAID-inducible COX it must be a conformational or structural variant. Potential mechanisms for variation would be alternative splicing, changes in posttranslational modification or differential interaction with intracellular proteins. Immunoblot analysis shows COX-2 in J774.2 cells undergoing NIA to be identical in size to COX-2 in the same cells induced by LPS. This finding argues against changes in glycosylation or phosphorylation states, which would alter electrophoretic mobilities. Moreover, by metabolic labelling and immunoprecipitation experiments we have shown that both COX-1 and COX-2 are unphosphorylated under the cellular states examined. This lack of phosphorylation is consistent with their intralumenal location within the endoplasmic reticulum, where the COX isoenzymes are likely shielded from cytosolic protein kinases. If alternative splicing occurs, it would have to produce a protein of the same size as native COX-2.

We have recently identified nucleobindin as a protein that interacts with cyclooxygenases in the yeast two hybrid system[17]. It is possible that signals mediated through this protein, which binds calcium and a proposed G protein, allosterically changes the structure of COX-2. A final possibility is that global changes in intracellular chemistry or membrane structure occurring during NIA expose COX-2 to a new intracellular milieu that radically changes its conformation and enzymatic properties. For example, glutathione, which is normally present at low concentration in the lumen of the ER but at high concentration in cytosol, has a particularly potent effect on both the COX catalytic rate and the profile of metabolic products of the enzyme[18]. Besides changing product profile, high glutathione levels in the presence of adrenaline also changes the reactivity of COX to paracetamol[19].

ALTERATION IN CHICKEN COX-2 PRE-mRNA SPLICING DURING NIA

In addition to being induced by virtually all NSAIDs that evoke NIA, the COX-2 mRNA is expressed as two species, 4.2 kb and 4.7 kb, during cell death (Figure 1). The 4.2 kb mRNA co-migrates with the fully processed COX-2 mRNA, and the 4.7 kb form with a partially processed mRNA in which intron 1 has been retained, as described previously[14,16]. COX-2 intron 1 has a unique structure not found in other introns. It contains a consensus 5' splice site but completely lacks a canonical 3' splice site. Additionally, 65% of the intron is composed of a unique repeat sequence not found elsewhere in the chicken genome. Splicing of this intron is exquisitely regulated, being accelerated by growth stimulating agents and inhibited by cellular quiescence or apoptosis. Thus this intron reflects a role of COX-2 in both of these processes. Sequences regulating the mitogen-induced splicing of this intron are located within the intron, whereas the sequences governing selection of the 3' splice site and inhibition of splicing are extra-intronic.

CHANGES IN CYTOSKELETAL PROTEINS, CELL CYCLE REGULATORS, AND SECRETORY FACTORS DURING NIA

Alterations in other potentially important proteins have been found, but their requirement for NIA has not been determined. Tissue transglutaminase, the level of which is elevated in many cell types undergoing apoptosis and which is necessary for crosslinking of cytoskeletal protein responsible for some morphological changes in the cell, is induced during NIA in CEF[14]. A secreted, quiescence-specific protein related to prostaglandin D2 synthase is specifically down-regulated during NIA in these cells[14]. DuBois and colleagues have also shown that E-cadherin is down-regulated during NIA in rat intestinal epithelial cells[10]. E-cadherin is an intrinsic cell surface protein that interacts with β-catenin, which is a substrate for pp60^{v-src}[20]. Like APC, which profoundly influences tumorigenesis of the colon, pp60^{c-src} shows elevated activity in colonic tumours at virtually all stages of progression[21]. Moreover, the APC protein, that regulates familial adenomatous polyposis in humans, binds to β-catenin[22]. Matings between mutant APC hemizygous mice and mice deficient in COX-2 produce progeny with greatly reduced polyp numbers and size. This effect could be mimicked by treatment of APC mutant mice with sulindac or MF tricyclic, a COX-2-selective NSAID[23]. These genetic and pharmacological data confirm the importance of COX-2 in tumorigenesis of the colon and suggest that inhibition of the cyclooxygenation site by NSAIDs can either prevent tumorigenesis by inhibiting cell division or by inducing apoptosis in the benign neoplasms. In other studies, administration of sulindac to humans and animals causes regression of pre-existing neoplasms, arguing for a direct role of apoptosis in this anti-tumorigenic effect. Further research will be needed to determine whether *src* and APC operate through the same signal transduction pathway to exert their effects on apoptosis governed by COX-2.

NIA IS NOT RESCUED BY COMMON COX PRODUCTS

If inhibition of COX-2 is necessary for NIA and the anti-tumorigenic effects of NSAIDs, are common prostaglandins synthesized from PGH_2 the cellular factors that maintain life in these cells? CEF make predominantly PGE_2 and small amounts of $PGF_{2\alpha}$. Neither of these prostaglandin isomers rescue CEF from NIA when applied to cells simultaneously with NSAID treatment. Concentrations tested ranged from 0.01 ng/ml to 10 µg/ml. Similar results were obtained with PGA_2 and PGD_2. At concentrations greater than 10 µg/ml these isomers instead caused apoptosis similar to that described for lymphocytes. However they were not as apoptotic as NSAIDs. These isomers plus a stable analog of PGI_2, PGJ_2, and $^{12}\Delta PGJ_2$ have been tested in mammalian cells, including J774.2 where they failed to rescue from NIA and where they also caused apoptosis at higher concentrations. PGG_2 and PGH_2 also failed to rescue from NIA, but were not lethal to cells even at concentrations above 10 µg/ml.

Recently Serhan and colleagues reported that the 15-(R)-HETE made by aspirin-acetylated COX-2 is synthesized by 5-lipoxygenase into bioactive 15-(R)-epilipoxin mediators[24]. Because these molecules are produced in the presence or absence of aspirin, and because NIA is aspirin insensitive, these compounds were of interest as possible mediators of NIA. We tested 15-(R)-HETE and five 15-(R)-epilipoxin isomers and found that they showed no signs of lethality, unlike prostaglandins (data not shown). However, they also did not rescue from NIA.

We have added large concentrations of potential fatty acid substrates to CEF in an attempt to partially block NIA, the concept being that at high concentration these fatty acids would effectively compete with NSAIDs. Arachidonic, linolenic, adrenic, oleic, and linoleic were non-toxic to cells up to concentrations of 125 µM. However, docosahexaenoic acid, eicosapentaenoic acid, dihomo-γ-lenolenic acid were toxic at concentrations above 200–300 µM. Docosahexaenoic acid is a competitive inhibitor of COX enzymes. Addition of these potential substrates failed to block NIA.

PGG_2 and PGH_2 both can undergo elimination of their cyclopentane ring to produce 12-(S)-hydroxy-heptadecatrienoic acid (12-(S)-HHT) and malondialdehyde. 12-(S)-HHT at concentrations up to 500 µg/ml was non-cytotoxic and did not inhibit

NIA. Malondialdehyde has not been tested but is known to be a physiologically important genotoxin and is expected to reduce cell growth by this mechanism[25].

The above data rule out an aspirin-inhibitable COX metabolite, such as currently known prostaglandins, as the biomediator that prevents apoptosis in these cells. Other metabolites, perhaps from shorter chain fatty-acids for which COX-2 has an isoenzymic preference, remain to be tested for preventing apoptosis.

DEFINING THE MOLECULAR TRIGGER OF NIA

Because the vast majority of NSAIDs cause apoptosis, and because the only shared pharmacological action of these drugs is inhibition of cyclooxygenase, where the structural mode of inhibition for NSAIDs is now defined at high resolution, we hypothesized that the event triggering NIA was the complete or near complete inhibition of one or more cyclooxygenases[14]. As described above, the preponderance of evidence suggests that this isoenzyme is COX-2. However, it is clear given the high NSAID doses needed for NIA, the ineffectiveness of aspirin in causing NIA, and the inability of prostaglandins to rescue cells from NIA, that the mechanism of action is not simple inhibition of prostaglandin synthesis.

Hanif et al. have recently identified NIA in several colon carcinoma cell lines[8]. They found that one of these, HCT-15 cells, lacked COX-1 and COX-2 mRNA. Therefore, they proposed NIA to be independent of either of these isoenzymes. We have tested this cell line for NIA and have found it to be sensitive to diclofenac, indomethacin and niflumic acid, in addition to the findings of Hanif et al. of sensitivity toward sulindac sulphide and piroxicam. HCT-15 cells were insensitive to apoptosis induced by aspirin, salicylate and paracetamol. Negligible amounts of PGE_2 were synthesized by this line in the presence or absence of exogenous arachidonic acid. Multiple analyses showed that PGE_2 levels were actually significantly lower than those in controls lacking any prostaglandins, suggesting that this line made a factor that interfered with the assay. Reverse transcription coupled polymerase chain reaction (RT-PCR) was therefore used to analyse for the COX-1 and COX-2 transcripts. No amplifiable COX-1 mRNA was found using two different primer pairs (data not shown). However, COX-2 primers readily amplified COX-2 cDNA (Figure 2). In comparable RT-PCR assays, COX-2 expression was found to be slightly lower than in another human colon carcinoma line (HT-29), and to be inducible by NSAID treatment (data not shown). These experiments support the concept that inhibition of COX-1 is unlikely to be the trigger of NIA, since these cells lack expression of that isoenzyme, but leave open the role of COX-2. The fact that only basal levels of COX-2 (similar to levels found in many cell types, including colonic epithelial cells) are present in HCT-15 cells would suggest that, if inhibition of COX-2 is the trigger initiating NIA, only small amounts of active COX-2 are needed to maintain cell life. This finding may explain why dexamethasone does not cause apoptosis even though it decreases expression of COX-2 mRNA by 70–80%[14]. This reduction may not reduce COX-2 past the critical minimum. High concentrations of competitive NSAIDs, on the other hand, may succeed in reducing COX-2 activity past this lethal threshold.

Not all cells are susceptible to NIA even though they express COX-2. A549 cells

Figure 2. RT-PCR amplification of COX-2 and β-actin cDNA in HCT-15 cells. 5 μg of HCT-15 or HT-29 poly (A) RNA was reverse transcribed using AMV reverse transcriptase (United States Biochemical) for 1 hour at 42°C. For human COX-2, primers were 5'-TTCAAATGAGATT-GTGGGAAAATTGCT-3' (a 27-mer sense oligonucleotide at position 573) and 5'-AGATCATCTCTGCCTGAGTATCTT-3' (a 24-mer antisense oligonucleotide at position 878), giving rise to a 303 bp PCR product. Human β-actin primers were 5'-GTTTGAGACCTTCAACACCCC-3' (1 21-mer sense oligonucleotide at position 409) and 5'-GTGGCCATCTCCTGCTCGAAGTC-3' (1 23-mer oligonucleotide at position 727), giving rise to a 318 bp PCR product. These were the same primers used by Hanif et al.[8]. PCR was performed for 40 cycles, using a cycling program of 94°C for 1 minute, 55°C for 1 minute, and 72°C for 1 minute. Following the amplification, an aliquot was loaded onto a 2% agarose gel. The third lane from the left contains poly (A) RNA isolated from HCT-15 cells that were treated for 40 hours with 500 μM diclofenac

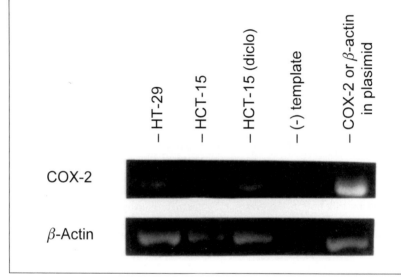

derived from a lung carcinoma are resistant to NIA even though COX-2 expression is highly induced by interleukin 1β treatment. The COX activity in these cells is very sensitive to inhibition by NSAIDs, demonstrating that resistance to NIA is not due to an inability of the drugs to permeate the cell membrane. Chronic treatment of these cells with NSAIDs not only does not induce cell death but also does not induce the NSAID-inducible COX activity described above. Resistance to NIA in these cells may indicate the expression of a dominant inhibitor of apoptosis, such as bcl-2. Or it may suggest that one or more effectors in the signalling pathway of NIA are missing.

Sulindac reduces tumorigenesis of the colon in animals and humans[26–28]. To act as an inhibitor of COX activity sulindac must first be metabolized in the liver or by intestinal flora to sulindac sulphide. Sulindac sulphide and sulindac sulphone, a metabolite that does not inhibit purified COX, are both inducers of apoptosis in mammalian colorectal cell lines. However, sulindac sulphide is 2–4 times more potent at causing cell death than is sulindac sulphone in these cells[9]. Given the ineffectiveness of sulindac sulphone at inhibiting COX activity, a logical conclusion from these data is that inhibition of COX-1 or -2 is not the trigger for NIA. However, our data above show an NSAID-inducible COX activity with distinctly different pharmacological properties from purified COXs. Thus an alternative hypothesis for the causation of apoptosis by sulindac sulphone, is that there is a cellular COX conformation that is inactivated by sulindac sulphone to initiate induction of apoptosis. This putative conformation variant is predicted to have an active site that differs from that in purified COX preparations.

Very recently, the PPARγ of the orphan steroid receptor class has been demonstrated to bind certain NSAIDs and to be activated by this binding[29]. This nuclear receptor promotes differentiation of some fibroblast-like cells into adipocytes. Another member of this transcription factor family, PPARα, also appears to be activated by NSAIDs. This receptor causes peroxisome proliferation and appears to promote cell division in hepatocytes. Initiators of peroxisome proliferation, such as clofibrate, both induce cell proliferation and COX-2 protein[30]. Interestingly, despite a large increase in COX-2, PGE_2 synthesis is unaltered or is decreased by these drugs. Thus the induced COX-2 is either catalytically inactive or it is making an unknown metabolite.

Our data show a strong qualitative correlation with the activation of the PPAR family and the induction of NIA. For example, indomethacin, flurbiprofen, and niflumic acid are all inducers of NIA and also activators of PPAR, whereas aspirin, salicylate and paracetamol are all inactive as inducers of NIA and as activators of PPAR. Furthermore, prostaglandins at high concentration are apoptotic. These eicosanoids activate PPAR and potentially could inhibit COX-2 through competition with arachidonic acid or mimicry of PGG_2.

NIA AND THE PREVENTION AND TREATMENT OF CANCER

The anti-neoplastic effects of NSAIDs may be multi-factorial. NSAIDs have been proposed to enhance natural killer cell activity by decreasing PGE_2 which is known to inhibit interleukin-mediated activation of lymphocytes. NSAIDs have also been shown to influence the cell cycle, and have been shown to arrest cell division[9]. Furthermore, in epidemiological and animal studies aspirin has been shown to reduce tumour incidence, although this compound is not a potent inducer of apoptosis. Thus, either through salicylate or by some indirect method this compound may exert its anti-tumorigenic effect.

The work of a number of laboratories, including our own, shows that competitively acting NSAIDs have a direct apoptotic effect on neoplastic cells, a mechanism by which these drugs potentially exert their anti-neoplastic effects in humans. At present, the data do not allow a simple inhibition of prostaglandin synthesis as the mechanism by which these drugs have a direct apoptotic effect. It is very possible that NIA is induced by the combined inhibition of COX-2 and the activation of a nuclear receptor, such as a member of the PPAR family. It has been theorized by others that the induction of COX-2 by peroxisome proliferating agents is to induce the growth response of these cells[30]. Presumably this would be through the synthesis of some metabolite. Because prostaglandin production does not increase following induction of COX-2 by PPAR agonists, this metabolite might be made from a non-arachidonic acid substrate or might be a novel arachidonate-derived compound. We speculate that the mixed message received by the cell to divide (from stimulation of a nuclear receptor) and to stop dividing (through inhibition of COX-2) results in a conflicting message which leads to apoptosis. Such a signalling conflict has been observed in the induction of cell death in many other cell types.

References

1. Kroemer G, Petit P, Zamzami N, Vayssiere J-L, Mignotte B. The biochemistry of programmed cell death. FASEB J. 1995; 9: 1277–87.
2. Mastino A, Piacentini M, Grelli S et al. Induction of apoptosis in thymocytes by prostaglandin E2 in vivo. Dev Immunol. 1992; 2: 263–71.
3. Brown DM, Warner GL, Ale-Martinez JE, Scott DW, Phipps RP. Prostaglandin E_2 induces apoptosis in immature normal and malignant B lymphocytes. Clin Immunol Immunopathol. 1992; 63: 221–9.
4. Abrahamsohn PA, Zorn TM. Implantation and decidualization in rodents. J Exp Zool. 1993; 266: 603–28.
5. Ackerman RC, Murdoch WJ. Prostaglandin-induced apoptosis of ovarian surface epithelial cells. Prostaglandins 1993; 45: 475–85.
6. Kim I-K, Lee J-H, Sohn H-W, Kim H-S, Kim S-H. Prostaglandin A_2 and Δ^{12}-prostaglandin J_2 induce apoptosis in L1210 cells. FEBS Lett. 1993; 321: 209–14.
7. Forman BM, Tontonoz P, Chen J, Brun RP, Spiegelman BM, Evans RM. 15-deoxy-$\Delta^{12,14}$-prostaglandin J_2 is a ligand for the adipocyte determination factor PPAR$_\gamma$. Cell. 1995; 83: 803–12.
8. Hanif R, Pittas A, Feng Y et al. Effects of nonsteroidal anti-inflammatory drugs on proliferation and on induction of apoptosis in colon cancer cells by a prostaglandin-independent pathway. Biochem Pharmacol. 1996; 52: 237–45.
9. Piazza GA, Rahm ALK, Krutzch M et al. Antineoplastic drugs sulindac sulfide and sulfone inhibit cell growth by inducing apoptosis. Cancer Res. 1995; 55: 3110–16.
10. Tsujii M, DuBois RN. Alterations in cellular adhesion and apoptosis in epithelial cells overexpressing prostaglandin endoperoxide synthase 2. Cell. 1995; 83: 493–501.
11. Elder DJE, Hague A, Hicks DJ, Paraskeva C. Differential growth inhibition by the aspirin metabolite salicylate in human colorectal tumor cell lines: Enhanced apoptosis in carcinoma and in vitro-transformed adenoma relative to adenoma cell lines. Cancer Res. 1996; 56: 2273–6.
12. Lu X, Fairbairn DW, Bradshaw WS, O'Neill KL, Ewert DL, Simmons DL. NSAID-induced apoptosis in Rous sarcoma virus-transformed chicken embryo fibroblasts is dependent on v-*src* and c-*myc* and is inhibited by *blc*-2. Manuscript submitted.
13. Thompson HJ, Jiang C, Lu J et al. Sulfone metabolite of sulindac inhibits mammary carcinogenesis. Cancer Res. 1997; 57: 267–71.
14. Lu X, Xie W, Reed D, Bradshaw WS, Simmons DL. Nonsteroidal antiinflammatory drugs cause apoptosis and induce cyclooxygenases in chicken embryo fibroblasts. Proc Natl Acad Sci USA. 1995; 92: 7961–5.
15. Holtzman MJ, Turk J, Shornick LP. Identification of a pharmacologically distinct prostaglandin H synthase in cultured epithelial cells. J Biol Chem. 1992; 267: 21438–45.
16. Xie W, Chipman JG, Robertson DL, Erikson RL, Simmons DL. Expression of a mitogen-responsive gene encoding prostaglandin synthase is regulated by mRNA splicing. Proc Natl Acad Sci USA. 1991; 88: 2692–6.
17. Ballif BA, Mincek NV, Barratt JT, Wilson MJ, Simmons DL Interaction of cyclooxygenases with an apoptosis- and autoimmunity-associated protein. Proc Natl Acad Sci USA. 1996; 93: 5544–9.

18. Jadwiga R, Wieckowski A, Gryglewski R. The effect of 4-acetamidophenol on prostaglandin synthetase activity in bovine and ram seminal vesicle microsomes. Biochem Pharmacol. 1978; 27: 393–6.
19. Smith WL, Marnett LJ. Prostaglandin endoperoxide synthase: structure and catalysis. Biochem Biophys Acta. 1991; 1083: 1–17.
20. Papkoff J. Regulation of complexed and free catenin pools by distinct mechanisms: Differential effects of Wnt-1 and v-*Src*. J Biol Chem. 1997; 272: 4536–43.
21. Talamonti MS, Roh MS, Curley SA, Gallick GE. Increase in activity and level of pp60[c-src] in progressive stages of human colorectal cancer. J Clin Invest. 1993; 91: 53–60.
22. Su LK, Vogelstein B, Kinszler KW. Association of the APC tumor suppressor protein with catenins. Science. 1992; 256: 668–70.
23. Oshima M, Dinchuk JE, Kargman SL et al. Suppression of intestinal polyposis in APC[Δ716] knockout mice by inhibition of cyclooxygenase 2 (COX-2). Cell. 1996; 87: 803–9.
24. Claria J, Serhan CN. Aspirin triggers previously undescribed bioactive eicosanoids by human endothelial cell–leukocyte interactions. Proc Natl Acad Sci USA. 1995; 92: 9475–9.
25. Chaudhary AK, Nokubo M, Reddy GR et al. Detection of endogenous malondialdehyde-deoxyguanosine adducts in human liver. Science. 1994; 265: 1580–2.
26. Labayle D, Fischer D, Vielh P et al. Sulindac causes regression of rectal polyps in familial adenomatous polyposis. Gastroenterology. 1991; 101: 635–9.
27. Thompson HJ, Jiang C, Lu J et al. Sulfone metabolite of sulindac inhibits mammary carcinogenesis. Cancer Res. 1997; 57: 267–71.
28. Boolbol SK, Dannenberg AJ, Chadurn et al. Cyclooxygenase-2 overexpression and tumor formation are blocked by sulindac in a murine model of familial adenomatous polyposis. Cancer Res. 1996; 56: 2556–60.
29. Lehmann JM, Lenhard JM, Oliver BB, Ringold GM, Kliewer SA. Peroxisome Proliferator-activated receptors α and γ are activated by indomethacin and other non-steroidal anti-inflammatory drugs. J Biol Chem. 1997; 272: 3406–10.
30. Ledwith BJ, Pauley CJ, Wagner LK, Rokos CL, Alberts DW, Manam S. Induction of cyclooxygenase-2 expression by peroxisome proliferators and non-tetradecanoylphorbol 12,13-myristate-type tumor promoters in immortalized mouse liver cells. J Biol Chem. 1997; 272: 3707–14.

6 Inhibition of intestinal tumorigenesis via selective inhibition of COX-2

R.N. DUBOIS, H. SHENG, J. SHAO, C. WILLIAMS and R. D. BEAUCHAMP

Clinical studies have shown a 40–50% reduction in relative risk of colorectal cancer in individuals taking aspirin on a regular basis [1–6]. Persons with familial adenomatous polyposis (FAP) who take sulindac show a striking reduction in adenoma size and number[7–11]. Since a potential target of these drugs is the cyclooxygenase (COX) enzymes, we set out to determine if COX-1 or -2 was dysregulated during the malignant transformation of intestinal epithelial cells.

We have previously reported increased COX-2 expression in human colorectal adenocarcinomas when compared to normal adjacent colonic mucosa[12]; these findings have been confirmed by other investigators who have shown elevated levels of COX-2 protein in colorectal tumours by Western blotting[13] and immunohistochemical staining[14]. We have also observed markedly elevated levels of COX-2 mRNA and protein in colonic tumours developing in rodents following carcinogen treatment[15] and in adenomas taken from *Min* mice[16]. Our observations of elevated COX-2 expression in three different models of colorectal carcinogenesis led us to consider the possibility that COX-2 expression may be related to colorectal tumorigenesis in a causal way. A recent study demonstrated a 40% reduction in aberrant crypt formation in carcinogen-treated rats who were given a selective COX-2 inhibitor[17]. Another study provided genetic evidence which directly links COX-2 expression to intestinal tumorigenesis in a mouse model[18,19]. In this study[19] APC$^{\Delta716}$ mice were generated which developed hundreds of tumours in their intestine. When these mice were bred with COX-2 null mice there was a 80–90% reduction in tumour multiplicity in the homozygous COX-2 null offspring. These results suggest that COX-2 may act as a tumour promoter in the intestine, and that increased levels of COX-2 expression may result directly from disruption of the APC gene.

To address the hypothesis that COX-2 is involved in colorectal tumorigenesis (Figure 1) we evaluated the growth of human colon cancer cells (HCA-7) that constitutively express COX-2 in nude mice with or without treatment with a highly selective COX-2 inhibitor (SC-58125)[20]. Additionally, we evaluated a colon cancer cell line (HCT-116) which lacks COX-2 expression to test for the selectivity of drug treatment.

Here we report that treatment with SC-58125 inhibits tumour growth by 85–90% in implanted HCA-7 cells which have high COX-2 expression but has no significant

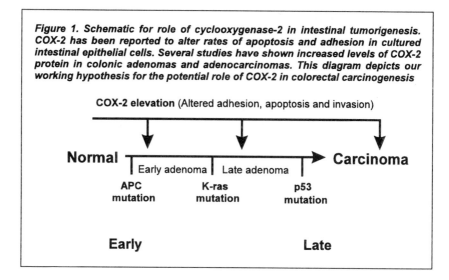

Figure 1. Schematic for role of cyclooxygenase-2 in intestinal tumorigenesis. COX-2 has been reported to alter rates of apoptosis and adhesion in cultured intestinal epithelial cells. Several studies have shown increased levels of COX-2 protein in colonic adenomas and adenocarcinomas. This diagram depicts our working hypothesis for the potential role of COX-2 in colorectal carcinogenesis

effect on implanted HCT-116 cells which lack COX-2 expression. These results suggest that COX-2 may be a feasible target for which to develop future agents for colon cancer prevention and treatment strategies.

MATERIALS AND METHODS

Prostaglandin (PG) measurements

Eicosanoids were quantified in media from cell incubations utilizing stable isotope dilution techniques employing gas chromatography/negative ion chemical ionization mass spectrometry as described[21,22]. The limits of sensitivity for detection of either PGE_2, PGD_2, $PGF_{2\alpha}$, or thromboxane B_2 and 6-ketoPGF$_{1\alpha}$ is 4 pg/ml.

Immunoblotting

Immunoblot analysis of cell protein lysates was performed as previously described[23]. Briefly, the cells were lysed for 30 minutes in RIPA buffer (1 × PBS, 1% Nonidet P40, 0.5% sodium deoxycholate, 0.1% SDS, 10 mg/ml) 0.1% then clarified cell lysates (100 μg) were denatured and fractionated by 12.5% SDS–PAGE. The proteins were transferred to nitrocellulose filters after electrophoresis, the filters were probed with an anti-human COX-2 antibody (Santa Cruz Biotechnology Inc., Santa Cruz, CA) and developed by the ECL chemiluminescence system (Amersham, Arlington Heights, IL) and exposed to XAR5 film (Kodak, New Haven, CT). Quantitation was carried out by video densitometry.

Tumour growth in nude mice

Cells suspended in 0.2 ml of DMEM medium were injected into the dorsal subcutaneous tissue of athymic nude mice (Sprague–Dawley nu/nu. Harlan). SC-58125 (10 mg/kg) was injected into peritoneal cavity of the mice prior to inoculation of cells. The treatment was continued 3 times a week at a dose of 5 mg/kg. Tumour volume was determined by external measurement according to published methods[24]. Volume was determined according to the equation ($V = [L \times W2] \times 0.5$, where V = Volume, L = Length, and W = Width).

RESULTS

Prostaglandin production

We measured PGE_2 production by HCA-7 and HCT-116 cells in both the presence and absence of SC-58125 (25 µM). The results, summarized in Table 1, indicated undetectable PGE_2 production in the HCT-116 cells, while PGE_2 production was significant in the HCA-7 cells (~10 ng/ml) and this was inhibited by SC-58125 treatment. Importantly, at the concentrations used in our study, SC-58125 has no inhibitory activity on COX-1[20].

Table 1. PGE_2 production in HCT-116 cells, and in HCA-7 cells in the presence or absence of the COX-2 selective inhibitor SC-58125

Cell line	PGE_2 (ng/ml)	SC-58125 (25 µM)
HCA-7	9.6	−
HCA-7	0.2	+
HCT-116	nd*	−
HCT-116	nd*	+

*nd = not detectable

Western blotting

The HCA-7 cells maintain high constitutive COX-2 expression, while the HCT-116 cells lack detectable COX-2 protein, although apparently some clones from this cell line have been reported to express low levels of COX-2 mRNA by PCR analysis[25]. We evaluated the effect of SC-58125 treatment on two established human colon cancer cell lines (HCA-7, colony 29 and HCT-116). The HCA-7 cell line was previously shown to constitutively express the COX-2 gene[22] which we confirmed by Western blot analysis. We evaluated another human colorectal cancer cell line (HCT-116) and found that it lacked expression of the COX-2 protein (Table 2).

Table 2. COX-2 expression in HCA-7 or HCT-116 cell lines. COX-2 is only expressed in HCA-7 cells. COX-1 is expressed in neither cell line

Cell line	COX-2 level	COX-1 level
HCA-7	++++	−
HCT-116	−	−

Selective inhibition of COX-2 inhibits solid tumour growth

We then evaluated the effect of SC-58125 on the growth of these two established human colon cancer cell lines (HCA-7 and HCT-116) when these cells were implanted as xenografts in nude mice. We first confirmed that both the HCA-7 and HCT-116 cell lines develop into solid tumours when implanted into nude mice (Table 3). Treatment of the nude mice with SC-58125 inhibited tumour development by 90% for the HCA-7 implants by day 7 but had no significant effect on implants of HCT-116 cells (Table 3). These experiments were conducted on 12 animals per time point for each group and have been reproduced in three separate sets of experiments. These data support the notion that SC-58125 inhibits tumour development of implants from COX-2 expressing colon cancer cells but not in cells that lack its expression and indicates that COX-2 activity may play a direct role in colorectal tumorigenesis in a set of colon cancers. The most important aspect of this experimental result is that it provides evidence for a link between COX-2 expression and responsiveness to selective inhibition of the COX-2 pathway.

Table 3. The effect of SC-58125 on tumour development in nude mice after xenografts of HCA-7 or HCT-116 cells. SC-58125 only inhibited tumour growth in the COX-2 expressing HCA-7 cells

Tumour xenograft	Size 100 mm³ (day 42)	SC-58125 (ip injection)
HCA-7	3.5	–
HCA-7	0.5	+
HCT-116	10.0	–
HCT-116	11.5	+

DISCUSSION

Recently, we reported that intestinal adenomas from *Min* mice express COX-2 mRNA and protein[16]. Since others have shown that tumour multiplicity is dramatically decreased in *Min* mice treated with non-steroid antiinflammatory drugs (NSAIDs)[26–28], our observation that COX-2 expression is elevated in early intestinal lesions from the *Min* mouse indicates that COX-2 may play a role early in tumorigenesis in this model. Numerous studies have reported that NSAIDs markedly reduce tumour burden in rats treated with the carcinogen azoxymethane, and one study indicates that selective COX-2 inhibition in these animals leads to a reduction in aberrant crypt formation[17]. We also found dramatically increased COX-2 levels in intestinal tumours which develop in azoxymethane-treated Fisher-344 rats[15], but COX-2 was absent in normal appearing intestinal mucosa from these animals. Thus, in two independent animal model systems for intestinal tumorigenesis, COX-2 is elevated early in the sequence of events leading to malignant transformation.

Because there is circumstantial evidence linking COX-2 expression to intestinal tumorigenesis, we set out to test the hypothesis that COX-2 is involved directly in intestinal tumour development (see Figure 1). In this study we chose to evaluate the response of two transformed intestinal epithelial cell lines to treatment with SC-58125, a selective COX-2 inhibitor. The HCA-7 cell line constitutively expresses the COX-2 gene. Treatment of HCA-7 cells with SC-58125 inhibited their growth as tumour implants in nude mice. The other cell line, HCT-116, lacks COX-2 expression and in these cells SC-58125 had no effect when they were implanted in nude mice. Other groups have reported effects of NSAIDs, used at very high concentrations, which are not likely to be due to their inhibition of COX enzymes[29]. Our result with the HCT-116 cells shows that SC-58125 is not acting as a non-specific cytostatic agent, but has a selective effect on transformed cells expressing COX-2.

Therapeutic relevance

Colorectal cancer is the second leading cause of cancer deaths in the US and the high mortality is due, in part, to the fact that by the time symptoms have developed the cancer has become metastatic. Currently, our best hope to reduce this high mortality is to develop better screening and prevention measures in order to detect the disease earlier or prevent it from developing. A new class of highly selective NSAIDs is currently being developed by pharmaceutical companies world-wide. These drugs, which include SC-58125 used here, are highly selective inhibitors of COX-2 and have little or no effect on COX-1 activity. In recent studies these drugs have been shown to have fewer side effects such as gastritis and ulcer disease, presumably due to their lack of COX-1 inhibition[20]. Because of their effectiveness in inhibiting growth of intestinal adenocarcinoma xenografts in mice, these agents may deserve a careful evaluation in patients at very high risk for colorectal cancer, such as persons with familial colon cancer syndromes and patients who have been previously treated for sporadic colorectal adenomas or cancer.

Acknowledgements

This work was supported in part by funds from the A.B. Hancock, Jr. Memorial Laboratory (RND), Lucille P. Markey Charitable Trust (RND) and the United States Public Health Services Grants NIHES 00267 (RND), DK 47297 (RND). RND is the recipient of a VA Research Associate career development award, Boehringer Ingelheim New Investigator Award, and is an AGA Industry Research Scholar.

References

1. Giovannucci E, Egan KM, Hunter DJ et al. Aspirin and the risk of colorectal cancer in women. N Eng J Med. 1995; 333: 609–14.
2. Greenberg ER, Baron JA, Freeman DHJ, Mandel JS, Haile R. Reduced risk of large-bowel adenomas among aspirin users. The Polyp Prevention Study Group. J Natl Cancer Inst. 1993; 85: 912–16.
3. Thun MJ, Namboodiri MM, Heath CWJ. Aspirin use and reduced risk of fatal colon cancer. N Engl J Med. 1991; 325: 1593–6.
4. Thun MJ, Namboodiri MM, Calle EE, Flanders WD, Heath CWJ. Aspirin use and risk of fatal cancer. Cancer Res. 1993; 53: 1322–7.
5. Peleg II, Maibach HT, Brown SH, Wilcox CM. Aspirin and nonsteroidal anti-inflammatory drug use and the risk of subsequent colorectal cancer. Arch Intern Med. 1994; 154: 394–9.
6. Giovannucci E, Rimm EB, Stampfer MJ, Colditz GA, Ascherio A, Willett WC. Aspirin use and the risk for colorectal cancer and adenoma in male health professionals. Ann Intern Med. 1994; 121: 241–6.
7. Giardiello FM, Hamilton SR, Krush AJ et al. Treatment of colonic and rectal adenomas with sulindac in familial adenomatous polyposis. N Engl J Med. 1993; 328: 1313–16.
8. Waddell WR, Loughry RW. Sulindac for polyposis of the colon. J Surg Oncol. 1983; 24: 83–7.

9. Waddell WR, Gasner GF, Cerise EJ, Loughry RW. Sulindac for polyposis of the colon. Am J Surg. 1989; 157: 175–8.

10. Winde G, Gumbinger HG, Osswald H, Kemper F, Bunte H. The NSAID sulindac reverses rectal adenomas in colectomized patients with familial adenomatous polyposis: clinical results of a dose-finding study on rectal sulindac administration. Int J Colorectal Dis. 1993; 8: 13–17.

11. Nugent KP, Farmer KC, Spigelman AD, Williams CB, Phillips RK. Randomized controlled trial of the effect of sulindac on duodenal and rectal polyposis and cell proliferation in patients with familial adenomatous polyposis. Br J Surg. 1993; 80: 1618–19.

12. Eberhart CE, Coffey RJ, Radhika A et al. Up-regulation of cyclooxygenase 2 gene expression in human colorectal adenomas and adenocarcinomas. Gastroenterology. 1994; 107: 1183–8.

13. Kargman S, O'Neill G, Vickers P, Evans J, Mancini J, Jothy S. Expression of prostaglandin G/H synthase-1 and -2 protein in human colon cancer. Cancer Res. 1995; 55: 2556–9.

14. Sano H, Kawahito Y, Wilder RL et al. Expression of cyclooxygenase-1 and -2 in human colorectal cancer. Cancer Res. 1995; 55: 3785–9.

15. DuBois RN, Radhika A, Reddy BS, Entingh AJ. Increased cyclooxygenase-2 levels in carcinogen-induced rat colonic tumors. Gastroenterology. 1996; 110: 1259–62.

16. Williams CW, Luongo C, Radhika A et al. Elevated cyclooxygenase-2 levels in *Min* mouse adenomas. Gastroenterology. 1996; 111: 1134–40.

17. Reddy BS, Rao CV, Siebert K. Evaluation of cyclooxygenase-2 inhibitor for potential chemopreventive properties in colon carcinogenesis. Cancer Res. 1996; 56: 4566–9.

18. Prescott SM, White RL. Self promotion? Intimate connections between APC and prostaglandin H synthase-2. Cell 1986; 87: 783–6.

19. Oshima M, Dinchuk JE, Kargman SL et al. Suppression of intestinal polyposis in APC$^{\Delta716}$ knockout mice by inhibition of prostaglandin endoperoxide synthase-2 (COX-2). Cell. 1996; 87: 803–9.

20. Masferrer JL, Zweifel BS, Manning PT et al. Selective inhibition of inducible cyclooxygenase-2 in vivo is antiinflammatory and nonulcerogenic. Proc Natl Acad Sci USA. 1994; 91: 3228–32.

21. DuBois RN, Awad J, Morrow J, Roberts LJ, Bishop PR. Regulation of eicosanoid production and mitogenesis in rat intestinal epithelial cells by transforming growth factor-α and phorbol ester. J Clin Invest. 1994; 93: 493–8.

22. Coffey RJ, Hawkey CJ, Damstrup L et al. EGF receptor activation induces nuclear targeting of COX-2, basolateral release of prostaglandins and mitogenesis in polarizing colon cancer cells. Proc Natl Acad Sci USA. 1997; 94: 657–62.

23. DuBois RN, Shao J, Sheng H, Tsujii M, Beauchamp RD. G$_1$ delay in intestinal epithelial cells overexpressing prostaglandin endoperoxide synthase-2. Cancer Res. 1996; 56: 733–7.

24. Wang J, Sun L, Myeroff L et al. Demonstration that mutation of the type II transforming growth factor beta receptor inactivates its tumour suppressor activity in replication error-positive colon carcinoma cells. J Biol Chem. 1995; 270: 22044–9.

25. Kutchera W, Jones DA, Matsunami N et al. Prostaglandin H synthase-2 is expressed abnormally in human colon cancer: Evidence for a transcriptional effect. Proc Natl Acad Sci USA. 1996; 93: 4816–20.

26. Beazer-Barclay Y, Levy DB, Moser AR et al. Sulindac suppresses tumorigenesis in the min mouse. Carcinogenesis. 1996; 17: 1757–60.

27. Jacoby RF, Marshall DJ, Newton MA et al. Chemoprevention of spontaneous intestinal adenomas in the Apc^{Min} mouse model by the nonsteroidal anti-inflammatory drug piroxicam. Cancer Res. 1996; 56: 710–14.

28. Boolbol SK, Dannenberg AJ, Chadburn A et al. Cyclooxygenase-2 overexpression and tumour formation are blocked by sulindac in a murine model of familial adenomatous polyposis. Cancer Res. 1996; 56: 2556–60.

29. Piazza GA, Rahm AL, Krutzsch M et al. Antineoplastic drugs sulindac sulfide and sulfone inhibit cell growth by inducing apoptosis. Cancer Res. 1995; 55: 3110–16.

7 Cyclooxygenase enzymes in human vascular disease

C. PATRONO, F. CIPOLLONE, G. RENDA, P. PATRIGNANI

The aim of this chapter is to review the involvement of cyclooxygenase (COX) isozymes in platelet–vessel wall interactions as well as to discuss the clinical implications of selective COX inhibition in human vascular disease.

LOW-DOSE ASPIRIN AS A SELECTIVE INHIBITOR OF PLATELET COX-1

The clinical development of low-dose aspirin as an antiplatelet agent provides an interesting paradigm of selective inhibition of a COX isozyme. During this process, we have learned important lessons in the use of analytical tools for studying the dose-dependence and biochemical selectivity of cyclooxygenase inhibition in man as well as observing the clinical correlates of such selectivity. Relatively selective inhibition of platelet COX-1 can be achieved by virtue of the irreversible inactivation of the enzyme and the very short half-life of aspirin in the human circulation (15–20 minutes). A 24-hour dosing interval allows full recovery of COX-1 activity in nucleated cells, but causes cumulative inhibition of enzyme activity in anucleated platelets upon repeated daily dosing with very low doses of the drug [1–3]. The unique mechanism of permanent inactivation of COX-1 by aspirin involves acetylation of a single amino acid residue (Ser-529) within the polypeptide chain of the enzyme. The strategic position of Ser-529 in the so-called cyclooxygenase channel blocks access of arachidonic acid to the active site of the enzyme, as a consequence of its acetylation by aspirin. Because of the irreversible nature of this modification, cyclooxygenase activity can be restored only by new protein synthesis (occurring within a few hours in nucleated cells) or platelet turn-over (occurring over days).

Inhibition of COX-1-dependent platelet function may lead to excess bleeding as well as to prevention of thrombosis. The balance between the two depends critically upon the absolute thrombotic vs. haemorrhagic risk of the patient. Thus, in individuals at very low risk for vascular occlusion (e.g. 1% per year), a very small absolute benefit is offset by exposure of a very large number of healthy subjects to undue bleeding complications [4,5]. In contrast, in patients at high risk of cardiovascular or cerebrovascular complications (>5% per year), the substantial absolute benefit of aspirin prophylaxis clearly outweighs the risks.

Aspirin-induced gastrointestinal toxicity, as detected in randomized clinical trials, appears to be dose-related in the range 30–1300 mg daily [5]. This is based largely on indirect comparisons of different trials and on a limited number of randomized, direct comparisons of different aspirin doses. Such a dose–response relationship is thought to reflect at least two COX-1-dependent components, i.e. dose-dependent inhibition of COX-1 in the gastrointestinal mucosa and dose-independent (within the examined range of doses) inhibition of COX-1 in platelets. The COX activity of gastric mucosa lining cells, as reflected by the output of PGE_2 and PGI_2 in the gastric juice, is hardly affected after single oral dosing with 100 mg, while COX-1 activity in platelets is completely abolished. Thus, it is not surprising that the antithrombotic effect of aspirin can be dissociated, at least in part, from its most common side-effects. However, even when administered at low doses, aspirin can cause serious gastrointestinal bleeding, as reported in studies using 30–50 mg daily. Because of the underlying prevalence of gastric mucosal erosions related to concurrent use of other non-steroidal anti-inflammatory drugs (NSAIDs), *Helicobacter pylori* infection and/or cigarette smoking, it is not surprising that any antiplatelet dose of aspirin will cause more bleeding from pre-existing lesions than a placebo. Low-dose aspirin has not been reported to affect renal function or blood pressure control[6], consistent with its lack of effect on renal prostaglandin synthesis[7].

Preliminary experience with selective COX-2 inhibitors, such as MK-966 and celecoxib, indicates that analgesic and antiinflammatory doses of these compounds do not affect platelet function in healthy subjects (see the chapters by Ford-Hutchinson and Needleman for details). Whether these novel agents may interfere with the acetylation of platelet COX-1 by aspirin, remains to be established.

TRANSCELLULAR INDUCTION OF ENDOTHELIAL COX-2 BY BIOACTIVE LIPIDS IN PLATELET MICROPARTICLES

Microparticles, or fragments of the plasma membrane, may be shed into the extracellular space following platelet activation, as result of an exocytotic budding process[8]. Both pro- and anti-coagulant activities have been detected in platelet microparticles[9], and circulating platelet-derived microparticles have been reported in syndromes of platelet activation, such as unstable angina[10]. Barry et al.[11] have recently characterized a novel mechanism for cellular activation by platelet microparticles which involves concentrated delivery of arachidonic acid to adjacent platelets and endothelial cells. Platelet activation requires prior metabolism of microparticle arachidonic acid to thromboxane (TX) A_2[11]. Interestingly, platelet microparticles could also induce expression of COX-2 and prostaglandin (PG)I_2 production, but not expression of COX-1, in human endothelial cells[11]. These effects were prevented by pretreatment with protein synthesis inhibitors, while microparticle-induced PGI_2 synthesis was reduced by a selective COX-2 inhibitor[11]. Expression of COX-2 was induced by the microparticle arachidonate fraction through a mechanism that did not involve activation of TXA_2, platelet activating factor or alpha-adrenoceptors[11]. Arachidonate in the platelet microparticles may serve as a substrate for the induced endothelial enzyme, contributing to enhanced PGI_2 formation. Although both PGE_2 and PGI_2 could evoke endothelial COX-2 expression at high concentrations, their kinetics differed from the response to platelet microparticles suggesting a direct effect of arachidonic acid on gene induction[11]. These studies suggest a novel mechanism by which the consequences of platelet activation may be modulated by a counter-regulatory induction of vascular PGI_2 synthesis, over an extended time-frame outlasting the short-term response involving the constitutive COX-1. Such a mechanism is consistent with an earlier demonstration of persistently enhanced PGI_2 formation in vivo, as reflected by elevated levels of its major urinary metabolite 2,3-dinor-6-keto-$PGF_{1\alpha}$, in clinical syndromes of platelet activation[12].

In contrast to a previously characterized mechanism of transcellular metabolism, involving platelet-derived PGH_2 to feed endothelial PGI_2 synthase[13], this novel modality of transcellular activation of endothelial cells involving the arachidonate fraction of platelet microparticles would be likely to operate in patients treated with low-dose aspirin and may, in fact, contribute to the biochemical selectivity of low-dose aspirin, in vivo, despite ex vivo evidence of inhibited endothelial COX-1 activity[14]. It is likely that the different turn-over rate of COX-1 vs. COX-2 as well as the differential aspirin sensitivity of the two isozymes may account for the biochemical selectivity of low-dose aspirin (Table 1). The effects of selective COX-2 inhibitors on this homeostatic mechanism of endothelial activation remain to be explored.

Table 1. Modalities and inhibitor susceptibility of endothelial PGI_2 production

Modality	Susceptibility to inhibition by	
	Low-dose aspirin	COX-2 Inhibitors
Constitutive	Yes	No
Inducible	No	Yes
Transcellular		
from platelet PGH_2	Yes	No
from platelet microparticles	No	Yes

ASPIRIN-RESISTANT TXA_2 BIOSYNTHESIS

Episodic increases in TXA_2 biosynthesis, as reflected by the urinary excretion of its major enzymatic metabolites, have been reported in patients with unstable angina[15-17]. Enhanced TXA_2 biosynthesis in this setting is likely to reflect episodes of platelet activation, because it was largely suppressed by low-dose aspirin[17]. However, despite >95% suppression of platelet COX activity by aspirin, as monitored ex vivo, incomplete suppression of 11-dehydro-TXB_2 excretion has been detected in some patients with unstable angina[17]. This finding prompted us to examine the hypothesis that a component of enhanced TXA_2 biosynthesis in unstable angina is dependent on the COX activity of nucleated cells, either insensitive to low-dose aspirin or rapidly recovering enzyme activity after aspirin acetylation by virtue of de novo enzyme synthesis[18]. Thus, we contrasted the biochemical effects of the short-lived aspirin with those of a long-lived, reversible COX inhibitor, indobufen, in a randomized, double-blind study of patients with unstable angina.

Indobufen is a reversible inhibitor of platelet COX activity[19]. When administered at a dose of 200 mg bid to patients recovering after myocardial infarction, indobufen suppressed platelet TXA_2 biosynthesis measured ex vivo by >95% throughout the dosing inverval[20]. Moreover, in patients with type-II diabetes mellitus, who are characterized by persistently elevated levels of TXA_2 biosynthesis[21], the same regimen of indobufen caused profound suppression of TXA_2 metabolite excretion[22], comparable to that achieved by low-dose aspirin in the same setting[21].

We randomized patients with unstable angina to a short-term treatment with either indobufen (200 mg bid) or aspirin (320 mg once daily) and collected consecutive urine samples up to 48 hours after randomization. The rationale for collecting as many as 18 urine samples from the same patient is related to the episodic nature of platelet activation and enhanced TXA_2 metabolite excretion, as previously characterized in unstable angina[15–17]. The main finding of this study was that the rate of TXA_2 biosynthesis was approximately 50% lower in patients treated with indobufen than in patients treated with aspirin[18].

Moreover, a significantly lower proportion of episodes of enhanced TXA_2 metabolite excretion was noted in association with indobufen as compared to aspirin (6 vs. 21%, respectively). Such a difference was not influenced by previous aspirin use, number of ischaemic episodes or invasive procedures during the study. The difference in TXA_2 metabolite excretion became apparent after the second daily dose of indobufen and persisted throughout the study[18].

As for the mechanism(s) underlying the different effects of aspirin and indobufen in suppressing TXA_2 biosynthesis, at least two alternative explanations might be considered. Firstly, the difference may have reflected incomplete inhibition of platelet COX activity by aspirin during the first two days of oral dosing. However, this seems unlikely because: (a) 320 mg causes a ceiling inhibitory effect on platelet COX activity; (b) the difference in 11-dehydro-TXB_2 excretion was also apparent in patients who had been exposed to aspirin prior to randomization to aspirin or indobufen; and (c) the episodes of enhanced metabolite excretion while on aspirin were uniformly distributed throughout the sampling period. Alternatively, the lower rate of TXA_2 biosynthesis while on indobufen may have reflected the inhibition by this drug of extra-platelet sources of TXA_2 biosynthesis, largely unaffected by aspirin because of rapid de novo synthesis of the enzyme in nucleated cells during the 24-hour dosing interval. Cells endowed with substantial amounts of TXA_2-synthase include monocyte/macrophages and, to a lesser extent, vascular cells[23]. The COX activity of monocyte COX-2 can be inhibited by high concentrations of aspirin that cannot be achieved after oral dosing with 320 mg, and by low, micromolar concentrations of indobufen compatible with the reported plasma levels of the drug after oral dosing with 200 mg bid. The catalytic activity of COX-2 might contribute to aspirin-insensitive TXA_2 biosynthesis by two distinct mechanisms (Table 2), i.e. by generating the intermediate PGH_2 as a substrate for

Table 2. Modalities and inhibitor susceptibility of TXA_2 production

Modality (cell type)	Susceptibility to inhibition by	
	Low-dose aspirin	COX-2 inhibitors
Constitutive (platelet)	Yes	No
Inducible (monocyte)	No	Yes
Transcellular (endothelial cell + platelet)	No	Yes

the TXA_2-synthase of the same cell (e.g. monocyte/macrophages) or through transcellular metabolism by providing exogenous PGH_2 to the TXA_2-synthase of aspirinated platelets[24]. The failure of indobufen to prevent completely episodes of increased TXA_2 biosynthesis may have reflected the relatively limited potency of the drug in inhibiting human monocyte COX-2, and/or less than maximal plasma levels of the drug during the first 24 hours, when all such episodes occurred. Thus, given the 8-hour half-life of the drug, steady-state plasma levels would not be achieved until the second day of twice daily dosing.

Despite obvious limitations, we believe that our findings might have some clinical as well as research implications. Aspirin-insensitive TXA_2 biosynthesis might provide a mechanism for the episodic formation of a potent agonist of the platelet and vascular TXA_2 receptors, possibly contributing to a number of clinical aspirin failures. The availability of potent and long-lasting TXA_2 receptor antagonists and selective COX-2 inhibitors offers the opportunity to test this hypothesis.

CONCLUSIONS

Although no studies have yet examined the impact of selective COX-2 inhibitors on the actual rate of TXA_2 biosynthesis in clinical syndromes of platelet activation, it is likely that these compounds will not effect COX-1-dependent platelet activation in vivo, based on the preliminary results of ex vivo measurements of platelet aggregation described elsewhere in this volume. Besides the obvious safety implications, this may also be relevant to long-term studies of selective COX-2 inhibitors vs. aspirin for the prevention of colorectal cancer, having mortality as an end-point.

The recently characterized transcellular activation of endothelial cells by bioactive lipids in platelet microparticles suggests the involvement of endothelial COX-2 in the sustained enhancement of PGI_2 production in response to persistent platelet activation. Whether attenuation of this potential homeostatic mechanism by selective COX-2 inhibitors will result in appreciable untoward consequences remains to be established.

Finally, the availability of selective COX-2 inhibitors may provide interesting tools to examine the pathophysiological significance of COX-2 induction in unstable coronary syndromes.

Acknowledgements

The expert editorial assistance of Andre Harris is gratefully acknowledged.

References

1. Burch JW, Stanford N, Majerus PW. Inhibition of platelet prostaglandin synthetase by oral aspirin. J Clin Invest. 1978; 61: 314–19.
2. Patrignani P, Filabozzi P, Patrono C. Selective cumulative inhibition of platelet thromboxane production by low-dose aspirin in healthy subjects. J Clin Invest. 1982; 69: 1366–72.
3. FitzGerald GA, Oates JA, Hawiger J et al. Endogenous biosynthesis of prostacyclin and thromboxane and platelet function during chronic administration of aspirin therapy in man. J Clin Invest. 1983; 71: 676–88.

4. Antiplatelet Trialists' Collaboration. Collaborative overview of randomised trials of antiplatelet therapy – I: prevention of death, myocardial infarction, and stroke by prolonged antiplatelet treatment in various categories of patients. Br Med J. 1994; 308: 81–106.
5. Patrono C. Aspirin as an antiplatelet drug. N Engl J Med. 1994; 330: 1287–94.
6. Mené P, Pugliese F, Patrono C. The effects of nonsteroidal anti-inflammatory drugs on human hypertensive vascular disease. Semin Nephrol. 1995; 15: 244–52.
7. Pierucci A, Simonetti BM, Pecci G et al. Improvement of renal function with selective thromboxane antagonism in lupus nephritis. N Engl J Med. 1989; 320: 421–5.
8. George JN, Pickett EB, Saucerman S et al. Platelet surface glycoproteins: Studies on resting and activated platelets and platelet membrane microparticles in normal subjects, and observations in patients during adult respiratory distress syndrome and cardiac surgery. J Clin Invest. 1986; 78: 340–8.
9. Tans G, Rosing J, Christella M et al. Comparison of anticoagulant and procoagulant activities of stimulated platelets and platelet-derived microparticles. Blood. 1991; 77: 2641–8.
10. Singh N, Gemmell CH, Daly PA, Yeo EL. Elevated platelet-derived microparticle levels during unstable angina. Can J Cardiol. 1995; 11: 1015–21.
11. Barry OP, Patricò D, Lawson JA, FitzGerald GA. Transcellular activation of platelets and endothelial cells by bioactive lipids in platelet microparticles. J Clin Invest. 1997; 99: 2118–27.
12. FitzGerald GA, Smith B, Pedersen AK, Brash AR. Increased prostacyclin biosynthesis in patients with severe atherosclerosis and platelet activation. N Engl J Med. 1984; 310: 1065–8.
13. Marcus AJ, Weksler BB, Jaffe EA, Broekman MJ. Synthesis of prostacyclin from platelet-derived endoperoxides by cultured human endothelial cells. J Clin Invest. 1980; 66: 9797–806.
14. Weksler BB, Pett SB, Alonso D et al. Differential inhibition by aspirin of vascular and platelet prostaglandin synthesis in atherosclerotic patients. N Engl J Med. 1983; 308: 800–5.
15. Fitzgerald DJ, Roy L, Catella F, FitzGerald GA. Platelet activation in unstable coronary disease. N Engl J Med. 1986; 315: 983–9.
16. Hamm CW, Lorenz RL, Bleifeld W, Kupper W, Weber W, Weber PC. Biochemical evidence of platelet activation in patients with unstable angina. J Am Coll Cardiol. 1987; 10: 988–1004.
17. Vejar M, Fragasso G, Hackett D et al. Dissociation of platelet activation and spontaneous myocardial ischemia in unstable angina. Thromb Haemostas. 1990; 63: 163–8.
18. Cipollone F, Patrignani P, Greco A et al. Differential suppression of thromboxane biosynthesis by indobufen and aspirin in patients with unstable angina. Circulation. 1997; 96: 1109–16.
19. Patrignani P, Volpi D, Ferrario R, Romanzini L, Di Somma M, Patrono C. Effects of racemic, S- and R-indobufen on cyclooxygenase and lipoxygenase activities in human whole blood. Eur J Pharmacol. 1990; 191: 83–8.
20. Rebuzzi AG, Natale A, Bianchi C, Mariello F, Coppola E, Ciabattoni G. Effects of indobufen on platelet thromboxane B_2 production in patients with myocardial infarction. Eur J Clin Pharmacol. 1990; 39: 99–100.
21. Davì G, Catalano I, Averna M et al. Thromboxane biosynthesis and platelet function in type II diabetes mellitus. N Engl J Med. 1990; 322: 1769–74.
22. Davì G, Patrono C, Catalano I et al. Inhibition of thromboxane biosynthesis and platelet function by indobufen in type II diabetes mellitus. Arterioscler Thromb. 1993; 13: 1346–9.
23. Nursing R, Ullrich V. Immunoquantification of thromboxane synthase in human tissues. Eicosanoids. 1990; 3: 175–80.
24. Karim S, Habib A, Lévy-Toledano S, Maclouf J. Cyclooxygenase-1 and -2 of endothelial cells utilize exogenous or endogenous arachidonic acid for transcellular production of thromboxane. J Biol Chem. 1996; 271: 12042–8.

8 Gastrointestinal effects of NSAIDs

C.J. HAWKEY

It is now one hundred years since Felix Hoffman first synthesized aspirin by acetylating salicylic acid[1]. This manoeuvre resulted in a molecule that caused less dyspepsia than the parent compound[2]. Aspirin proved highly effective as an analgesic and as an anti-inflammatory agent and has become the world's most successful drug. Because aspirin was given to patients with rheumatic fever, it was initially feared that it might be cardiotoxic[1], but this has turned out to be spurious guilt by association. However, sporadic observations that aspirin was gastrotoxic were formally confirmed in 1937 when endoscopic studies clearly showed it caused haemorrhages, erosions and ulcers in the gastric mucosa[3].

The realization that aspirin was gastrotoxic stimulated developments in the analgesic field. Paracetamol had been devised about the same time as aspirin but been less popular partly because of fears that it might share the toxicity of phenacetin, and partly because it was manifestly less effective. With the realization that paracetamol did not damage the gastric mucosa, its popularity grew in the post-war era. The desire for a compound as effective as aspirin but without its toxicity stimulated development of a second wave of aspirin like drugs – the non-aspirin non-steroid anti-inflammatory drugs (NSAIDs): approximately 20 different NSAIDs were released between 1960 and 1990.

Unfortunately, non-aspirin NSAIDs were not an advance in terms of toxicity. Indeed, the growing popularity of these drugs since the mid-1960s has been paralleled by a rise in the incidence of ulcer complications, particularly in elderly women[4]. Substantial data now show a causal role for NSAIDs, though they may not fully account for the magnitude of the rise[5,6]. Whilst an increasing prevalence of *H. pylori* in elderly patients could also be an important factor, there may be other unidentified causes.

A number of early observations suggested that there may be two or more isoforms of the cyclooxygenase (COX) enzyme which results in prostaglandin synthesis and whose activity is inhibited by NSAIDs[7-9]. These observations have been confirmed by the identification of the constitutive COX-1 enzyme responsible for housekeeping functions such as platelet aggregation and gastro-protection[10] and the COX-2 enzyme, inducible at sites of inflammation by a wide variety of stimuli and suppressible by corticosteroids[11]. In consequence, a third generation of aspirin-like drugs with the potential for reduced gastrotoxicity are under evaluation. Meloxicam, a relatively selective COX-2 inhibitor is already available[12]. Highly selective COX-2 inhibitors are in phase III trials.

SPECTRUM OF NSAID ASSOCIATED GASTROINTESTINAL INJURY

Oesophageal injury

The relationship between NSAID use and oesophagitis is a vexed and unanswered one. Patient studies suggest that NSAID users have an increased risk of benign oesophageal stricture, a consequence of oesophagitis[13]. However, most prostaglandins relax the gastrooesophageal junction and in some studies NSAIDs have been shown to increase lower oesophageal tone, thus abrogating one of the main risk factors for gastro-oesophageal reflux disease[14]. Moreover, in some animal models NSAIDs have been protective to the oesophageal mucosa[15]. If NSAIDs are harmful to the oesophageal mucosa, this may arise indirectly: NSAID use appears to be associated with secretion of epidermal growth factor into saliva[16].

Gastroduodenal injury

Numerically the bulk of NSAID toxicity in humans falls on the gastroduodenal mucosa. Acute macroscopic gastric mucosal injury is near universal following aspirin ingestion but less common with single doses of non-aspirin NSAID[17,18]. However, approximately 20% of chronic NSAID users have an endoscopically evident ulcer in the stomach or duodenum and risks of ulcer complications and death are increased 3- to 10-fold[6].

One important characteristic of NSAID-associated ulcers is that they are frequently silent, with very little dyspepsia prior to presentation with an ulcer complication. Equally, although acetylation of salicylate to produce aspirin reduced the high levels of dyspepsia seen with non-acetylated salicylates, there is still a substantial level of dyspepsia associated with aspirin and non-aspirin NSAID use[19]. These two observations make the use of dyspepsia to predict the presence of NSAID-associated ulcers almost useless. Levels of dyspepsia bear a significant relationship to the extent of mucosal prostaglandin synthesis, consistent with a facilitatory role for prostaglandins in the perception of dyspeptic (and other) pain[20]. It seems therefore that both the improved tolerability of aspirin relative to salicylic acid and the increased toxicity may both be attributable to the ability of aspirin and non-aspirin NSAIDs to inhibit prostaglandin synthesis.

Relationship between NSAIDs and *Helicobacter pylori*

This is a controversial area with many conflicting data in the literature[21]. Acute studies of the damaging effects of NSAIDs in subjects infected by and free of *H. pylori* have been inconclusive. Some have shown increased acute injury with *H. pylori* whilst others have shown no difference. None has shown protection. Likewise, endoscopic studies of the prevalence of ulcers in NSAID users have either found no effect or increased numbers of ulcers in those infected with *H. pylori*. However, these studies can be criticized since nearly all have studied patients presenting for endoscopy for clinical indications[21]. These studies have therefore included a disproportionate number of NSAID users with dyspepsia. All studies that have investigated the question directly have shown that NSAID-associated dyspepsia is more common in subjects infected with *H. pylori* than those not infected. By inducing gastric inflammation, *H. pylori* enhances prostaglandin synthesis and the higher level of dyspepsia in infected patients can be related to this partial abrogation of the normal reduction caused by NSAIDs[20,22].

Studies of ulcer complications have consistently shown no significant interaction, either additive or synergistic between NSAID use and *H. pylori*[23,24]. Thus, in one study[23] NSAID use was the main factor associated with peptic ulcer bleeding and co-existence of *H. pylori* only increased risk by 1.1-fold.

If the two main causes of peptic ulcer, acting by different mechanisms do not have even additive effects on the risk of ulcer complications, one possibility is that the intrinsic toxicity of one is counter-balanced by cross protection against the other. It is plausible that the ability of *H. pylori* to abrogate the reduction in prostaglandin synthesis associated with NSAID use may protect against ulceration to an extent roughly equal to its own ability to cause ulcer disease. If this hypothesis is true, one would predict that where the ulcerogenic efects of *H. pylori* are prevented (by use of acid suppression) benefits to NSAID users of being infected by *H. pylori* should become apparent. Recent studies of the influence of *H. pylori* in NSAID users taking omeprazole or ranitidine have confirmed this prediction. When taking the acid suppressing drugs ranitidine or omeprazole (but not misoprostol), NSAID users infected with *H. pylori* had faster ulcer healing and reduced relapse rates compared to those who were *H. pylori*-negative[25,26].

Intestinal lesions

In rats, the burden of toxicity with indomethacin is in the small intestine rather than the stomach or duodenum. These animals die from multiple small intestinal ulcers often with secondary infection. In these animals an intact enterohepatic circulation is required for toxicity and protection can be achieved with antibiotics[27]. In recent years, it has become clear that small intestinal ulceration is also a feature of NSAID use in humans. A postmortem study showed a 5–10% prevalence of small intestinal ulceration in patients taking NSAIDs prior to death[28]. These studies have been substantiated by enteroscopic studies[28]. Epidemiological studies show a more than two-fold increase in the risk of small and large intestinal perforation[29]. A rare but specific complication of NSAID use is the development of valve-like lesions resulting in pinhole lumen obstruction of the small intestine and high mortality[30].

For some time, NSAID use has been associated with exacerbation of ulcerative colitis. There have been grounds to believe that this might be consequential rather than causal, since a similar association has been shown for paracetamol usage[31]. However, recent studies strongly suggest a causal role for NSAIDs in development or relapse of ulcerative colitis[32]. One possible interpretation of the association with paracetamol use is therefore that this too is acutely causal, with the implication that paracetamol might, in the colon, show some of the toxicity of NSAIDs.

Preventing the gastrointestinal side effects of NSAIDs

The upper gastrointestinal side effects of NSAIDs can be avoided by non-use or (probably) by switching to paracetamol[33]. Epidemiological studies have consistently shown that ibuprofen is the least toxic of the current NSAIDs in major use[34]. Switching to ibuprofen is therefore likely to reduce the burden of ulcer disease[34]. The reduced toxicity of ibuprofen may largely reflect its reduced potency but it is a short-acting NSAID which persists in the joint for longer than in the plasma[35] resulting in an enhancement of its therapeutic benefit relative to its harmful effects. Moreover, the analgesic, as opposed to the anti-inflammatory, effects of NSAIDs appear to reach asymptotic levels at relatively low doses[36]. Thus use of low doses and/or ibuprofen may genuinely reduce toxicity more than they reduce therapeutic benefits.

Other important risk factors for ulcer complications are old age, past history, co-administration of steroids and co-administration of warfarin. Patients with these risk factors needing to take significant doses of NSAIDs may require protection by co-therapy. Two choices are available: prostaglandin 'replacement' with misoprostol[37], or acid peptic protection with omeprazole[25,26] or high dose famotidine[38].

Numerous studies have shown misoprostol reduces acute mucosal injury and endoscopically evident ulcers[39] and, in one large study, the need for hospital admission with ulcer complications[37]. Normal doses of H_2 antagonists can prevent endoscopically evident duodenal ulcers but do not have a significant effect on gastric ulceration[39]. However, recent data with high doses of famotidine and with omeprazole show that greater elevation of the pH, probably to around 4, is protective against acute mucosal injury[40,41], and both gastric and duodenal ulcers in endoscopic studies[25,26,28].

In comparative trials, omeprazole 20 mg daily has been shown to be as effective as misoprostol 200 μg qds for healing ulcers or multiple erosions, more effective than misoprostol 200 μg bd for maintenance, better tolerated than misoprostol and more effective than ranitidine 150 mg bd for both healing and maintenance[25,26]. In these studies, omeprazole healed gastric and duodenal ulcers significantly faster than misoprostol, and there was a reduced incidence of ulcer at relapse. Conversely, misoprostol was more effective in healing multiple erosions and there was a reduced incidence of erosions at relapse compared to omeprazole. In all these studies, there was a strong correlation between the site and nature of the initial lesion and that seen at relapse, suggesting that the increased risk of ulcer disease in patients with a past history was due to local mucosal rather than general factors.

Gastrointestinal cancer

An interesting observation is that colonic cancers over-express COX-2. A growing body of epidemiological data suggest that patients who consume aspirin have a reduced risk of fatal GI cancer[42]. Follow-up studies of patients who have undergone colonoscopy have also shown a reduced development of colorectal adenomas after a negative colonoscopy and reduced recurrence in those with an initial positive colonoscopy[43]. More limited data also suggest that these observations may extend to at least some of the non-aspirin NSAIDs and to other gastrointestinal cancers[42].

Many questions remain to be answered. The precise distribution within tumours of COX-2 is controversial, as is the mechanism by which COX-2 leads to enhanced malignant transformation. Aspirin is an incomplete inhibitor of the COX-2 enzyme which alters the profile of products of arachidonic acid metabolism. Whether more complete highly selective COX-2 inhibitors will be more or less effective than aspirin is an important question that remains to be determined.

OVERALL BENEFITS OF NSAIDs

Whilst much attention has focused on the hazards of aspirin and NSAID use, a risk/benefit analysis suggests that for aspirin at least the benefits far outweigh the hazards[44]. This analysis suggests that daily use of aspirin 300 mg from age 30 to death has the potential to result in a reduction per 100 000 white male users of 1166 for colorectal cancer, 6120 for myocardial infarction, with an increase of only 28 gastrointestinal bleeds. Certainly, no study has ever shown an overall reduction in life expectancy in NSAID users. Indeed in one study overall life expectancy was (non-significantly) increased and there was a significant increase in the life expectancy of one subgroup largely attributable to reduced cardiovascular events[45].

Thus, in the 100 years since aspirin was first synthesized, there have probably been net benefits to its use and that of non-aspirin NSAIDs. With the advent of highly specific COX-2 inhibitors, the second century of NSAIDs and the gut is likely to be as interesting as the first.

References

1. Mann CC, Plummer ML. The Aspirin Wars, Money, Medicine, and 100 years of Rampant Competition. Boston: Harvard Business School Press, 1991.
2. Insel PA. Analgesic-antipyretics and anti-inflammatory agents: Drugs employed in the treatment of rheumatoid arthritis and gout. In: Goodman Gilman A, Rall TW, Nies AS, Taylor P (eds). Goodman & Gilman's The Pharmacological Basis of Therapeutics. 8th edition New York: Pergamon Press; 1990.
3. Douthwaite A, Lintott CA. Gastroscopic observations of the effect of aspirin and certain other substances on the stomach. Lancet. 1938; 2: 1222.
4. Walt R, Katschinski B, Logan R, Ashley J, Langman MJS. Rising frequency of ulcer perforation in elderly people in the United Kingdom. Lancet. 1986; I: 489–92.
5. Hawkey CJ. Non-steroidal anti-inflammatory drugs and ulcers: Facts and figures multiply, but do they add up? Br Med J. 1990; 300: 278–84.
6. Henry D, Robertson J. Non steroidal anti-inflammatory drugs and peptic ulcer hospitalization rates in New South Wales. Gastroenterology. 1993; 104: 1083–91.
7. Morrison ARK, Nishikawa K, Needleman P. Thromboxane A_2 biosynthesis in the ureter obstructed isolated perfused kidney of the rabbit. J Pharmacol Exp Ther. 1978; 205: 1–8.
8. Hawkey CJ, Truelove SC. Effect of prednisolone on prostaglandin synthesis by rectal mucosa in ulcerative colitis. Gut. 1981; 22: 190–3.
9. Fuj Y, Masferrer JL, Seibert K, Raz A, Needleman P. Induction and suppression of prostaglandin H2 synthase (cyclooxygenase) in human monocytes. J Biol Chem. 1990; 265: 1–4.
10. Kujubu DA, Fletcher BS, Varnum BC, Lim RW, Herschman HR. TIS10, a phorbol ester tumour promoter-inducible mRNA from Swiss 3T3 cells, encodes a novel prostaglandin synthase/cyclooxygenase homologue. J Biol Chem. 1991; 266: 12866–72.
11. Masferrer JL, Zweifel BS, Manning PT et al. Selective inhibition of inducible cyclooxygenase 2 in vivo is anti-inflammatory and non ulcerogenic. Proc Natl Acad Sci USA. 1994; 91: 3228–32.
12. Hawkey CJ, Längström G, Naesdal J, Yeomans ND. Significance of dyspeptic symptoms during healing and maintenance of NSAID-associated gastroduodenal lesions with omeprazole, misoprostol and ranitidine. Lancet. 1997 (submitted).

13. Heller SR, Fellows IW, Ogilvie AL, Atkinson M. Non steroidal anti-inflammatory drugs and benign oesophageal stricture. Br Med J. 1985; 285: 167–8.

14. Scheiman JM, Patel PM, Henson EK, Nostrant TT. Effect of naproxen on gastroesophageal reflux and oesophageal function: A randomised, double-blind, placebo-controlled study. Am J Gastroenterol. 1995; 90: 754–7.

15. Northway MG, Castell DO. Do prostaglandins cause gastrointestinal mucosal injury? Dig Dis Sci. 1981; 26: 453–6.

16. Jones PDE, Daneshmend TK, Bossingham DH, Swannell AJ, Doherty M, Hawkey CJ. Reduced production of salivary epidermal growth factor in rheumatoid patients. Eur J Gastroenterol Hepatol. 1990; 2: 203–7.

17. Hawkey CJ, Hawthorne AB, Hudson N, Cole AT, Mahida YR, Daneshmend TK. Separation of aspirin's impairment of haemostasis from mucosal injury in the human stomach. Clin Sci. 1991; 81: 565–73.

18. Hawkey CJ, O'Morain C, Murray FE, McCarthy C, Tiernay D, Devane J. Two comparative endoscopic evaluations of naprelan. Am J Orthopedics. 1996; 25: 30–6.

19. Rampton DS, McNeil NI, Sarner M. Analgesic ingestion and other factors preceding relapse in ulcerative colitis. Gut. 1983; 24: 187–9.

20. Hudson N, Balsitis M, Everitt S, Hawkey CJ. Enhanced gastric mucosal leukotriene B_4 synthesis in patients taking non-steroidal anti-inflammatory drugs. Gut. 1993; 34: 742–7.

21. Hawkey CJ. Are NSAIDs and *Helicobacter pylori* separate risk factors. In: Hunt Rh, Tytgat GNJ (eds). *Helicobacter pylori*, Basic Mechanisms to Clinical Cure 1996. Dordrecht: Kluwer Academic Publishers, 1996: 312–23.

22. Cullen DJE, Hull MA, Hudson N et al. Dyspepsia with non-steroidal anti-inflammatory drugs: Role of prostaglandins and enteric neurones. Proceedings of the Midlands Gastroenterological Society; 1994.

23. Cullen DJE, Hawkey GM, Greenwood DC et al. Peptic ulcer bleeding in the elderly: Relative roles of *Helicobacter pylori* and non steroidal anti inflammatory drugs. Gut. 1996 (submitted).

24. Labenz L, Köhl H, Wolters S et al. *Helicobacter pylori*, NSAIDs and the risk of peptic ulcer bleeding – a prospective case-control study with matched pairs. Gastroenterology. 1996: 110: A165.

25. Hawkey CJ, Swannell AJ, Yeomans ND, Langstrom G, Lofberg I, Taure E. Site specific ulcer relapse in non steroidal anti inflammatory drug (NSAID) users: Improved prognosis with *H. pylori* and with omeprazole compared to misoprostol. Gut. 1996; 39: A149.

26. Hawkey CJ, Swannell AJ, Yomans ND, Carlsson M, Floren I, Jallinder M. Increased effectiveness of omeprazole compared to ranitidine in non steroidal anti inflammatory drug (NSAID) users with reference to *H. pylori* status. Gut. 1996; 39: A149.

27. Satoh H, Inada I, Hirata T, Maki Y. Indomethacin produces gastric antral ulcers in the refed rat. Gastroenterology. 1981; 81: 719–25.

28. Allison MC, Howatson AG, Torrance CJ, Lee FD, Russell RI. Gastrointestinal damage associated with the use of non steroidal anti inflammatory drugs. N Eng J Med. 1992; 327: 749–54.

29. Langman MJS, Morgan L, Worral A. Use of anti-inflammatory drugs by patients admitted with small or large bowel perforation and haemorrhage. Br Med J. 1985; 290: 347–9.

30. Bjarnason I, Price AB, Zanelli G. Clinicopathological features of non steroidal anti-inflammatory drug induced small intestinal strictures. Gastroenterology. 1988; 94: 1070–4.

31. Rampton DS, McNeil NI, Sarner M. Analgesic ingestion and other factors preceding relapse in ulcerative colitis. Gut. 1983; 24: 187–9.

32. MacDonald TM. Side effects of non steroidal anti-inflammatory drugs: Studies from the Tayside medicines monitoring unit. Inflammopharmacology. 1995; 3: 321–6.

33. Maynard A, Bloor K. Is there scope for improving the cost-effective prescribing of non steroidal anti-inflammatory drugs. PharmacoEconomics. 1996; 6: 484–96.

34. Henry D, Lim LL-Y, Garcia Rodriguez LA et al. Variability in risk of gastrointestinal complications with individual non-steroidal anti-inflammatory drugs: results of a collaborative meta-analysis. Br Med J. 1996; 312: 1563–6.

35. Brooks P, Day RO. Non steroidal anti-inflammatory drugs – differences and similarities. N Eng J Med. 1991; 324: 1716–25.

36. Gotzsche PC. Methodology and overt and hidden bias in reports of 196 double-blind trials of non steroidal anti-inflammatory drugs in rheumatoid arthritis. Controlled Clin Trials. 1989; 10: 31–56.
37. Silverstein FE, Graham DY, Senior JR et al. Misoprostol reduces serious gastrointestinal complications in patients with rheumatoid arthritis receiving non steroidal anti-inflammatory drugs – a randomised double blind placebo controlled study. Ann Intern Med. 1995; 123: 241–9.
38. Taha A, Hudson N, Hawkey CJ et al. Famotidine for prevention of gastric and duodenal ulcers caused by non steroidal anti inflammatory drugs. N Eng J Med. 1996; 334: 1435–9.
39. Koch M, Dezi A, Ferrario F, Capurso L. Prevention of non steroidal anti-inflammatory drug induced gastrointestinal mucosal injury: A meta-analysis of randomised controlled clinical trials. Arch Intern Med. 1996; 156: 2321–31.
40. Daneshmend TK, Pritchard J, Bhaskar NK, Millns P, Hawkey CJ. Use of microbleeding and an ultrathin endoscope to assess gastric mucosal protection by famotidine. Gastroenterology. 1989; 97: 944–9.
41. Daneshmend TK, Stein AG, Bhaskar NK, Hawkey CJ. Abolition by omeprazole of aspirin induced gastric mucosal injury in humans. Gut. 1990; 31: 514–17.
42. Thun MJ, Namboodiri MM, Calle EE, Flanders WD, Heath CW Jr. Aspirin use and risk of fatal cancer. Cancer Res. 1993; 53: 1322–7.
43. Rex DK, Cummings OW, Helper DJ et al. 5-year incidence of adenomas after negative colonoscopy in asymptomatic average-risk persons. Gastroenterology. 1996; 111: 1178–81.
44. Russo MW, Helm JF, Simpson KN, Ransohoff DF, Wurzelmann JI, Sandler RS. Weighing the benefits and risks of low-dose aspirin in primary prevention of colorectal cancer (CRC). Gastroenterology. 1996; 110: A36.
45. Guess HA, West R, Strand LM et al. Fatal upper gastrointestinal haemorrhage or perforation among users and non users of non steroidal anti-inflammatory drugs in Saskatchewan, Canada 1983. J Clin Epidemiol. 1988; 41: 35–45.

9 Renal side effects of NSAIDs: role of COX-1 and COX-2

J. C. FRÖLICH and D. O. STICHTENOTH

NSAIDs are widely prescribed and are also available as over-the-counter drugs. Thus, a large number of patients are exposed. Renal failure due to NSAID accounted for approximately 6% of all patients with the disease observed in a 2-year period[1]. In a prospective study by Kleinknecht et al. NSAID caused 16% of drug induced acute renal failure and 3% of all acute renal failure[2]. Recent observations on patients with end-stage renal failure implicated NSAIDs as causal agents in 30% of cases[3].

The unwanted renal effects of NSAIDs can be divided into 3 categories: (1) renal side effects of NSAID due to inhibition of prostaglandin (PG) synthesis. Most of the unwanted renal effects of NSAID are related to this mechanism, including reduction in renal blood flow (RBF), glomerular filtration rate (GFR), sodium retention and hyperkalaemia[4,5]. (2) Interstitial nephritis: this can be caused by many drugs which are not NSAIDs such as the ß-lactam antibiotics. The disease usually requires months of drug exposure and it has been suggested that it is a cell mediated immune response[2]. (3) Analgesic nephropathy, a condition characterized by a slowly developing process that begins in the papilla and later involves the vasa recta. The lesions are characterized by cell death leading to characteristic papillary necrosis which is characterized as an ischaemic necrosis due to medullary ischaemia[6]. The end result is loss of ability to concentrate urine, papillary calcification and loss of papillae. Many different factors have been involved in the causation of the damage including concentration of the offending agent due to the counter current mechanism, exhaustion of GSH due to the formation of reactive drug metabolites and reduction in medullary perfusion, which, due to low oxygen tension in this tissue easily leads to ischaemic damage[5].

ORIGIN AND ASSESSMENT OF RENAL PROSTAGLANDINS

In vitro studies showed that the whole cortex or medulla could produce PGE_2, $PGF_{2\alpha}$ and PGI_2[7,8]. These studies led to the proposal that PGI_2 is primarily synthesized in the cortex and PGE_2 in the medulla[9]. While this has generally held true, some exceptions were noted depending on the experimental conditions[10]. More detailed analyses of isolated structures of the kidney have shown that the renal vasculature and glomeruli produce mainly PGI_2, while renomedullary interstitial cells synthesize predominantly PGE_2[11,12]. There is also some thromboxane A_2 (TXA_2) synthesis; the functional role of this, however, is uncertain[9].

One of the substantial challenges has been to analyse renal PG production in vivo. Blood levels of PGs are unreliable parameters due to platelet activation and irritation of the vascular wall[13]. It is also technically difficult to obtain samples from the renal artery and veins, particularly when repeat sampling is necessary. All of these problems are compounded when studies in humans are performed.

In contrast, urinary PGE_2 excretion is a valid, non-invasive index parameter for renal PG production. However, there are some limitations. In males, seminal fluid may interfere with PGE_2 measurements, as it contains about 25–50 µg/ml PGE_2 while the 24 hour excretion in females is only about 200 ng[13,14]. Furthermore, PG excretion may depend on pH as PGs are weak acids. In fact, Haylor et al. showed, that alkalinization of urine increased, and acidification decreased, urinary PG excretion[15]. A further complication is the urine flow rate: there is some reabsorption of PGs which is reduced when the flow rate is increased[16]. In summary, measurement of urinary PGE_2 in females provides a good index of renal PG production in humans[17]. This parameter has been used extensively to delineate the physiological and pathophysiological role of PGs and is very useful to assess drug effects on the kidney as will be shown below.

PHYSIOLOGICAL ACTIONS OF PGs IN THE KIDNEY AND EFFECTS OF NSAID

Regulation of renal haemodynamics

The first evidence for an effect of PGs on renal blood flow stems from infusion of PGE_1 into a renal artery of dogs which produced an increase in RBF[18]. Other PGs, including PGE_2, PGD_2 and PGI_2, were also shown to cause an increase in RBF[19]. There are also vasoconstrictor responses to PGE_2, but these disappear or are converted to vasodilation by antagonists of angiotensin II[20], which suggests that the observed vasoconstriction is secondary to renin release.

Inhibition of cyclooxygenase (COX) by indomethacin in experiments in anaesthetized, laparatomized dogs showed striking reductions of RBF and led to the proposal that PGs are responsible for regulation of basal RBF[21]. However, in later studies in conscious dogs indomethacin had no effect on RBF[22,23]. This difference points to the important role of other mediators (catecholamines, angiotensin II, vasopressin) which, when unopposed by renal PGs, cause pronounced vasoconstriction. A wealth of information has now accumulated to suggest that in pathophysiological states PGs help to maintain RBF and GFR. This is particularly true for those disorders characterized by a low effective plasma volume: cirrhosis with ascites, heart failure and the nephrotic syndrome, where vasoconstrictor effects of renal nerve activity, catecholamines, angiotensin II and vasopressin play an important role. Accordingly, indomethacin causing a striking decrease in GFR in patients with nephrotic syndrome[24], congestive heart failure[25] and liver cirrhosis[26].

There are other conditions in which the underlying mechanism is not so apparent, in which inhibition of PG synthesis also reduces GFR including Bartters' Syndrome[27], chronic renal insufficiency[28], SLE with renal involvement[29] and sodium depletion due to diet or use of diuretics[30]. Under these conditions the effect of PG synthesis inhibition may become very severe and induce acute renal failure.

There is a further effect of renal PG inhibition with far-reaching consequences:

medullary blood flow is provided exclusively by the juxtamedullary nephrons. These nephrons are the only source of arterial blood for the medulla. PG synthesis inhibition will affect the distribution of blood flow within the kidney away from the medulla[31]. Thus, PGs play a critical role in protecting the renal medulla from ischaemic damage[32]. This may be one important contributory factor to papillary necrosis caused by the currently used NSAIDs[4].

Electrolyte excretion

Sodium

Infusion of arachidonic acid or PGE_2 causes natriuresis[18]. This effect is coupled with vasodilation and this may be the cause of the natriuresis presumably by an effect on proximal tubular salt and water reabsorption. However, there is also evidence that tubular transport is influenced by PGs directly. Indomethacin and meclofenamate were shown to enhance sodium reabsorption at a point beyond the proximal tubule[33]. Later studies showed that chloride also was affected and, further, that during volume expansion, reabsorption of electrolytes was inhibited in the thick ascending limb by meclofenamate[34]. Direct evidence supporting a tubular action of PGE_2 on sodium reabsorption stems from microinfusions of ^{22}Na into the distal proximal tubule. This study shows that co-infusion of PGE_2 reduces Na reabsorption[33]. Studies in isolated renal tubular segments showed that PGE_2 inhibits sodium transport out of the cortical collecting tubule, thus suggesting a direct inhibitory effect of PGE_2 on sodium transport[35]. From these studies it can be deduced that PGs, most likely PGE_2, reduce sodium reabsorption in a segment beyond the proximal tubule. This PG-dependent natriuresis occurs primarily in the juxtamedullary nephrons[36]. Accordingly, meclofenamate has been shown to enhance sodium reabsorption particularly by this mechanism of enhanced absorption in the juxtamedullary nephrons[34]. The role of antidiuretic hormone (ADH, vasopressin) on sodium transport is perhaps underestimated. PGs antagonize ADH actions (see later) and the inhibition of ADH-enhanced sodium transport by PGE_2 contributes to the effects of PGs on sodium excretion.

In humans the evidence of a sodium-retaining effect following PG suppression is quite firm, when the appropriate parameters (sodium intake, urine excretion, body weight) have been thoroughly controlled. Of particular importance is the fact, that sodium retention will only occur for a brief period in most cases and a new steady state will be reached within a few days. We were able to show that in patients with post-malignant hypertension in a 100 mEq Na^+ diet, indomethacin (25 mg t.i.d.) readily caused inhibition of renal PG production, sodium retention and weight gain[37].

In normal volunteers, sodium retention and weight gain are more difficult to demonstrate[37]. In contrast, in patients with nephrotic syndrome[24], congestive heart failure[25] and liver cirrhosis[26], sodium retention is readily observed after PG inhibition and may lead to significant clinical deterioration.

The simultaneous decrease of RBF/GFR and sodium excretion make it difficult to localize the site of action of the drugs. However, in most studies sodium retention is more severe than can be explained solely by a reduction in the filtered load and an increased tubular resorption is the only explanation.

Potassium

Potassium excretion can be reduced by NSAIDs. The increase in plasma potassium concentration is associated with, and probably caused by, a reduction in plasma renin activity (PRA). Inhibition of renal PG production by indomethacin or ibuprofen with lower PRA together with aldosterone, but increase sodium reabsorption[37]. Indomethacin will also completely abrogate the increase in plasma renin activity seen within minutes after giving furosemide intravenously to normal volunteers[37]. The lowering of aldosterone is not due to a direct effect of PG inhibition on aldosterone secretion from the adrenal because infusion of angiotensin II resulted in increases in aldosterone before and after indomethacin administration[37]. In sodium-depleted normal volunteers suppression of PRA by NSAIDs can only be observed under conditions of inhibited sympathetic drive of renin release by nonselective betareceptor blockade. Under these conditions, when sodium retention was eliminated by a low sodium diet renin release could be blocked by indomethacin[38]. Our further investigations showed, that the macula densa was responsible for PG mediated renin release[39]. The prostanoid most likely involved is PGI_2, because in contrast to PGE_2 we found it to be a potent releaser of renin from renal cortical slices[40].

Hyperkalaemia is not a common problem in patients with normal renal function but may become a severe threat to the patient with renal disease, which may by itself cause potassium retention, or when drugs which cause potassium retention are taken simultaneously.

Lithium

Effects of NSAIDs on plasma levels of lithium are described in several case reports. We studied this drug interaction in a controlled fashion and showed plasma lithium concentrations to increase with indomethacin and diclofenac[41,42]. This effect is due to a decrease in renal lithium clearance and has now been observed with other NSAIDs including oxyphenbutazone and ketoprofen. Interestingly, in a cross-over study in normal volunteers we observed a decrease in renal lithium clearance with diclofenac but no effect of aspirin in spite of a very similar reduction in renal PG production[43]. Salicylate has no effect on renal lithium clearance[44]. The reason for this anomalous behaviour of salicylate and aspirin is unknown[43]. From these examples for pronounced differences amongst the NSAIDs it becomes obvious that extrapolations between NSAIDs are not possible.

Antidiuretic hormone

Endogenous PGs attenuate the hydroosmotic effect of ADH[45]. This interaction takes place at the medullary site, where very large amounts of PGE_2 can be synthesized[46]. The first in vivo study to test the hypothesis that renal PGs antagonize the action of ADH was carried out in hypophysectomized dogs to prevent uncertainties about endogenous ADH production. Indomethacin or meclofenamate administration produced a powerful increase of urine osmolality in response to ADH[47] and it was suggested, that PGs function as negative feedback inhibitors of ADH action. In humans, infusion of hypertonic saline increases urine osmolality and free water reabsorption, and both effects are enhanced by indomethacin[48], showing that endogenous ADH, released in large amounts by hypertonic saline, will become more effective, when renal PG production is suppressed.

The type of PG involved was shown by systematic studies of various PGs. PGE_2 and PGF_2 exerted the greatest activity[49]. In cultured canine epithelial cells[50] or in canine cortical collecting tubule cells[12] PGE_2 was found to be the most potent antagonist of ADH action.

The mechanism of the interaction between ADH and PGs has been studied repeatedly. No convincing evidence has been forthcoming for an interaction on the level of cAMP but PGs could affect the intracellular calcium pool, which is required for ADH action[51]. In fact PGE_2 decreased the size of this store and thus could exert its antagonistic action by ADH by this mechanism[52]. PGs have a further effect which is intimately involved in water transport, i.e. the solute concentration of the renal papilla. PGs enhance renal and papillary blood flow and this causes a wash-out of the papillary concentration gradient[53]. In vivo studies support this concept as PG synthesis inhibitors enhance sodium and chloride concentrations in the renal medulla[54] and increase sodium reabsorption in Henle's loop[34].

It cannot be ascertained which of the above mechanisms of the ADH/PG antagonism are operative in vivo. However, from a functional point of view it is important to recognize that under the maximal influence of ADH virtually no barrier to water reabsorption exists in the collecting duct and there is complete equilibration with the medullary interstitium. Under these conditions inhibition of PG synthesis is still effective and enhances antidiuresis, thus an influence on water permeability alone cannot explain the findings.

DIFFERENCES BETWEEN EFFECTS OF NSAIDs ON RENAL FUNCTION

It has been generally accepted that NSAIDs act by inhibiting PG production by competitive or irreversible blockade of COX. The most often observed problem is that of a reduction in RBF and/or GFR as acute renal failure and the formation of oedema[4,5]. However, not all NSAIDs are alike. For example, paracetamol does not inhibit platelet aggregation and has a very weak effect on renal PG production in man[55]. Non-acetylated salicylates like salicylate, salsalate or diflunisal also show no effect on platelet aggregation, platelet thromboxane production or renal PGE_2 synthesis at dosages which are antiinflammatory in man[56]; the experience with patients suffering from unwanted effects of NSAIDs shows that these drugs do not cause sodium retention and oedema, reduction in renal blood flow and GFR, papillary necrosis, haematuria, water intoxication and hyperkalaemia[57,58]. Furthermore, glucocorticoids, which in vitro were effective in inhibiting PG production[59], were shown by us to have no effect on PG production in healthy animals[60] and normal volunteers even at dosages that induced a Cushing appearance[61].

SELECTIVE INHIBITION OF COX-2 AS NEW STRATEGY TO AVOID NSAID SIDE-EFFECTS

The discovery of two different forms of COX[62–64], now known as COX-1 and COX-2, has explained some of the differences between NSAID mentioned above and ushered in a new generation of NSAID with the promise of fewer side effects on the gastrointestinal tract and the kidney[65].

COX-1 is the constitutive enzyme serving the basic physiological functions mediated by PGs. These include regulation of peripheral vascular resistance, renal blood flow and GFR, renal sodium excretion, ADH-antagonism and possibly renin release. COX-2, which shows only 60% identity of its amino acid sequence with COX-1, is induced by interleukins and mitogens (IL-1, transforming growth factor ß, tumour necrosis factor α, endotoxin and fibroblast growth factors). It is induced in pregnancy in the uteroplacental unit and may well be the source of enhanced PG production in pregnancy. COX-2 can be induced in human monocytes, human synovial cells, chondrocytes and many other cell types, suggesting that in inflammatory reactions enhanced PG production is due to induction of COX-2. This makes COX-2 an outstanding target for therapeutic interventions[66].

What are the data on COX-1 and COX-2 in the kidney? COX-1 has been found in arteries and arterioles, glomeruli and collecting ducts. Remarkably, no COX-1 has been found in the proximal or distal convoluted tubule, Henle's loop or the macula densa[67]. COX-2 has been detected in low concentrations in the kidneys of victims of accidents but no localization has been given[68].

In a detailed analysis of the distribution of COX enzymes in the rat kidney Harris et al. reported that under control conditions some COX-2 is observed in the cortex, papilla and in medullary interstitial cells. That in the cortex is strikingly increased during long-term sodium depletion[69]. The major location of COX-2 was in the macula densa, which is important for the control of renin release. These findings were recently confirmed by Pairet et al. in vivo in rats[70]. Indomethacin, a preferential COX-1 inhibitor (see below), as well as the highly selective COX-2 inhibitor SC 58125, blocked the furosemide stimulated PRA in rats on low sodium diet. Thus, COX-2 may play a predominant role in the control of renin release in rat kidney. Interestingly, urinary PGE_2 excretion was markedly reduced by indomethacin but unaffected by SC 58125, suggesting that apart from the macula densa, renal PG production is COX-1 dependent in rats.

In man, experimental data suggest that under normal basal conditions COX-2 plays a minor role in the kidney. Glucocorticoids have a pronounced effect on PG production in diseased kidneys, yet they will not cause a deterioration of renal function. Because glucocorticoids inhibit the induction of COX-2[71], they should have detrimental effects on renal function, if COX-2 derived PGs were important in the kidney. However, this has never been shown. The sodium retention seen after glucocorticoid administration is due to their mineralocorticoid effect and not due to PG suppression. Our observation that furosemide-stimulated renin release in the first few minutes is completely abrogated in man by indomethacin suggests, that the renin release is due to a constitutive enzyme[37]. However, this issue remains open and needs further investigation.

The effect of NSAIDs on COX-1 and COX-2 has been investigated repeatedly under various experimental conditions. Biochemical studies in which COX-1 and COX-2 had been expressed in cells or cell membranes by transfection, or in which COX-2 was induced by endotoxin, showed inhibition of the enzymes with indomethacin and piroxicam, but these two drugs were more effective against COX-2, while ibuprofen and the active metabolite of nabumetone (6-MNA) were more effective against COX-2[72].

In another study comparing indomethacin and diclofenac, diclofenac was 10 times more powerful as an inhibitor of COX-2 relative to COX-1 than indomethacin[73]. While the species and the models varied considerably, the following trend emerges: indomethacin and piroxicam are particularly active on COX-1 while ibuprofen, diclofenac and 6-MNA are less active on COX-1. Paracetamol was without effect on COX-2 and had only a weak effect on COX-1[74]. Interestingly, salicylate was 20 times less effective than acetylsalicylic acid against COX-1 but only half as effective against COX-2, making it a relatively selective COX-2 inhibitor. On the basis of inhibition of platelet aggregation one could assume that non-acetylated salicylates are very weak COX-1 inhibitors[56].

NEW SELECTIVE COX-2 INHIBITORS

The prospect of finding an NSAID with selectivity for COX-2 which would have less gastric and renal toxicity has led to the development of numerous new drug candidates.

Meloxicam, which is marketed in some European countries since 1996, is a new COX-2 selective NSAID. The ratio of the IC_{50} values for inhibition of COX-1/COX-2 by meloxicam is, depending on the experimental model, in the range 100 to 3[75–77]. In a rat model of inflammation (carageenin pleurisy) meloxicam showed much more activity against inhibition of pleuritic than renal PG production and compared favourably in its selectivity to diclofenac, tenoxicam, tenidap, piroxicam and indomethacin[76].

We have performed a cross-over study of meloxicam 7.5 mg/day in 14 normal female volunteers comparing it to indomethacin in the equi-effective antiinflammatory dosage of 75 mg[78]. We found that indomethacin, but not meloxicam, caused a significant inhibition of arachidonate (1 mM)-induced platelet aggregation. Accordingly thromboxane B_2 formation in response to arachidonate was completely inhibited by indomethacin but remained unaffected by meloxicam. Because these parameters are exclusively COX-1 dependent, our results indicate a sparing of COX-1 by meloxicam and strong inhibition of this enzyme by indomethacin at the chosen dose level. Indomethacin reduced urinary PGE_2 excretion by about 50% while meloxicam did not show a significant reduction (Figure 1). Clinical studies in high-risk patients for developing renal failure will be needed to show whether this selectivity seen in normal volunteers translates into a renal sparing effect.

So far only preliminary data are available: a small study including 25 patients with mild renal impairment suggested that meloxicam 15 mg/d for 28 days did not cause further deterioration of renal function[79]. Initial reports on a total of 3727 patients in double blind clinical trials, showed that diclofenac caused an increase of serum creatinine to values >1.8 in 1.8% of those on piroxicam, and in 2% of those on

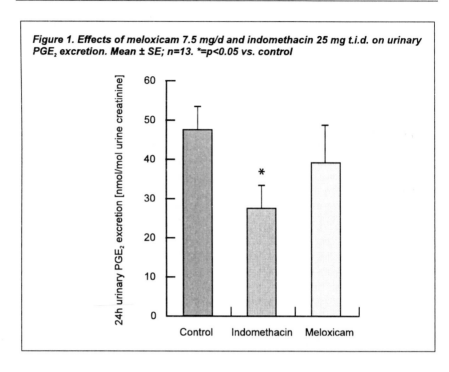

Figure 1. Effects of meloxicam 7.5 mg/d and indomethacin 25 mg t.i.d. on urinary PGE₂ excretion. Mean ± SE; n=13. *=p<0.05 vs. control

naproxen, but meloxicam produced this effect in 0.5 and 0.1% of patients on a dose of 15 or 7.5 mg respectively (data on file, Boehringer-Ingelheim). While this shows a much reduced risk of renal problems with meloxicam, it also shows that the drug will not be completely free of renal side effects.

Celecoxib (SC58635, Monsanto/Searle) and MK966 (Merck-Frosst), now tested in clinical trials, are highly selective COX-2 inhibitors with up to a 1000-fold greater selectivity for COX-2 than COX-1 in in vitro assays. The experiences with meloxicam suggest that highly selective COX-2 inhibitors would have significantly less renal and gastrointestinal side effects.

In summary, selective COX-2 inhibition holds the promise to provide drugs which will have significantly less unwanted effects on the kidney. These drugs would be expected not to cause reduction in GFR/RBF, medullary damage, sodium retention, possibly no hyperkalaemia and no interactions with antihypertensive drugs or lithium.

References

1. Corwin HG, Bonventre JV. Renal insufficiency associated with non-steroidal antiinflammatory agents. Am J Kidney Dis. 1984; 4: 147–52.
2. Kleinknecht D. Diseases of the kidney caused by non-steroidal antiinflammatory drugs. In: Stewart JH (ed.) Analgesic and NSAID-induced Kidney Disease. Oxford: Oxford University Press 1993: 160–79.

3. Schwarz A, Offermann G, Keller F. Analgesic nephropathy and renal transplantation. Nephrol Dial Transplant. 1992; 7: 427–32.
4. Whelton A, Hamilton CW. Nonsteroidal anti-inflammatory drugs: Effects on kidney function. J Clin Pharmacol. 1991; 31: 588–98.
5. Schlondorff D. Renal complications of nonsteroidal anti-inflammatory drugs. Kidney Int. 1993; 44: 643–53.
6. Nanra RS, Kincaid-Smith P. Experimental evidence for nephrotoxicity of analgesics. In: Stewart JH (ed). Analgesic and NSAID-induced kidney disease. Oxford: Oxford University Press 1993: 17–31.
7. Lee JB, Covino BJ, Takman GH, Smith ER. Renomedullary vasodepressor substance medullin: isolation, chemical characterization, and physiological properties. Circ Res. 1965; 17: 57–70.
8. Larsson C, Anggard E. Regional differences in the formation and metabolism of prostaglandins in the rabbit kidney. Eur J Pharmacol. 1973; 21: 30–6.
9. Whorton AR, Smigel M, Oates JA, Frölich JC. Regional differences in prostaglandin formation by the kidney: Prostacyclin is a major prostaglandin of renal cortex. Biochim Biophys Acta. 1978; 529: 176–80.
10. Hassid A, Dunn MJ. Biosynthesis and metabolism of prostaglandins in human kidney in vitro. In: Dunn MJ, Patrono C, Cinotti GA (ed). Prostaglandins and the kidney. New York: Plenum Press; 1982: 3–15.
11. Grenier FC, Rollins TE, Smith WL. Kinin-induced prostaglandin synthesis by renal papillary collecting tubule cells in culture. Am J Physiol. 1981; 241: 94–104.
12. Garcia-Perez A, Smith WL. Apical-basolateral membrane asymmetry in canine cortical collecting tubule cells: Bradykinin, arginine vasopressin, prostaglandin E_2 interrelationships. J Clin Invest. 1984; 74: 63–74.
13. Frölich JC. Methods in prostaglandin research, Raven, New York: 1979.
14. Patrono C, Wennmalm A, Ciabattoni G, Nowak J, Pugliese F, Cinotti GA. Evidence for an extra-renal origin of urinary prostaglandin E_2 in healthy men. Prostaglandins. 1979; 18: 623–9.
15. Haylor J, Lote CJ, Thewles A. Urinary pH as a determinant of prostaglandin E_2 excretion by the conscious rat. Clin Sci. 1984; 66: 675–81.
16. Frölich JC, Rosenkranz B, Fejes-Toth G, Naray-Fejes-Toth A, Frölich B. Analysis of prostanoid metabolites by gas chromatography-mass-spectrometry. Adv Prostaglandin, Thromboxane Leukotriene Res 1985, 15: 47–52.
17. Frölich JC, Wilson TW, Sweetman BJ et al. Urinary prostaglandins. Identification and origin. J Clin Invest. 1975; 55: 763–70.
18. Johnston HH, Herzog JP, Lauler DP. Effect of prostaglandin E_1 on renal hemodynamics, sodium and water excretion. Am J Physiol. 1967; 213: 939–46.
19. Lifschitz MD. Prostaglandins and renal blood flow. Kidney Int. 1981; 19: 781–5.
20. Schör N, Brenner BM. Possible mechanism of prostaglandin-induced renal vasoconstriction in the rat. Hypertension. 1981; 3(suppl II): 81–5.
21. Aiken JW, Vane JR. Intrarenal prostaglandin release attenuates the renal vasoconstrictor activity of angiotensin. J Pharmacol Exp Ther. 1973; 184: 678–87.
22. Swain JA, Heyndrickx GB, Borttcher DH, Vatner SF. Prostaglandin control of renal circulation in the unanesthetized dog and baboon. Am J Physiol. 1975; 229: 826–30.
23. Kirschenbaum MA, Stein JH. Effect of inhibition of prostaglandin synthesis on urinary sodium excretion in conscious dog. J Clin Invest. 1976; 57: 517–21.
24. Arisz L, Donker AJM, Brentjens JRH, van der Hem GK. The effect of indomethacin on proteinuria and kidney function in the nephrotic syndrome. Acta Med Scand. 1976; 199: 121–5.
25. Walshe JJ, Venuto RC. Acute oliguric renal failure induced by indomethacin: Possible mechanism. Ann Intern Med. 1979; 91: 47–9.
26. Antillon M, Cominelli F, Lo S et al. Effects of oral prostaglandins on indomethacin induced renal failure in patients with cirrhosis and ascites. J Rheumatol. 1990; 17: 46–9.
27. Gill JR, Frölich JC, Bowden RE et al. Bartter's syndrome, a disorder characterized by high urinary prostaglandins and a dependence of hyperreninemia on prostaglandin synthesis. Am J Med. 1976; 61: 43–51.

28. Berg, KJ. Acute effects of acetylsalicylic acid in patients with chronic renal insufficiency. Eur J Clin Pharmacol. 1977; 11: 111–16.
29. Kimberley RP, Gill JR, Bowden RE, Keiser HR, Plotz PH. Elevated urinary prostaglandins and the effects of aspirin on renal function in lupus erythematosus. Ann Intern Med. 1978; 89: 336–41.
30. Frölich JC, Brill AB, Oates JA. Reduced GFR associated with decreased prostaglandin synthesis produced by indomethacin in sodium deprived humans. Clin Res. 1975; 23: 373A.
31. Itskovitz HD, Terragno NA, McGiff JC. Effect of a renal prostaglandin on distribution of blood flow in the isolated canine kidney. Circ Res. 1974; 34: 770–6.
32. Brezis M, Rosen S. Hypoxia of the renal medulla – its implications for disease. N Engl J Med. 1995; 332: 647–55.
33. Kauker ML. Prostaglandin E_2 effect from the luminal side on renal tubular ^{22}Na efflux: Tracer microinjection studies. Proc Soc Exp Biol Med. 1977; 154: 274–7.
34. Higashihara E, Stokes JB, Kokko JP, Campbell WB, Du Bose TD Jr. Cortical and papillary micropuncture examination of chloride transport in segments of the rat kidney during inhibition of prostaglandin production: A possible role of prostaglandins in the chloruresis of acute volume expansion. J Clin Invest. 1979; 64: 1277–87.
35. Stokes JB, Kokko JP. Inhibition of sodium transport by prostaglandin E_2 across the isolated, perfused rabbit collecting tubule. J Clin Invest. 1977; 59: 1099–104.
36. Stokes JB. Effect of prostaglandin E_2 on chloride transport across the rabbit thick ascending limb of Henle, selective inhibition of the medullary portion. J Clin Invest. 1979; 64: 495–502.
37. Frölich JC, Hollifield JW, Dormois BL et al. Suppression of plasma renin activity by indomethacin in man. Circ Res. 1976; 39: 447–52.
38. Frölich JC, Hollifield JW, Michelakis AM et al. Reduction of plasma renin activity by inhibition of the fatty acid cyclooxygenase in human subjects: Independence of sodium retention. Circ Res. 1979; 44: 781–7.
39. Data JL, Gerber JG, Crump WJ, Frölich JC, Hollifield JW, Nies AS. The prostaglandin system: A role in canine baroreceptor control of renin release. Circ Res. 1978; 42: 454–8.
40. Whorton AR, Misono K, Hollifield J, Frölich JC, Inagami T, Oates JA. Prostaglandins and renin release: I. Stimulation of renin release from rabbit renal cortical slices by PGI_2. Prostaglandins. 1977; 14: 1095–104.
41. Frölich JC, Leftwich R, Ragheb M, Oates JA, Reimann I, Buchanan D. Indomethacin increases plasma lithium. Br Med J. 1979; 1: 1115–16.
42. Reimann IW, Frölich JC. Effects of diclofenac on lithium kinetics. Clin Pharmacol Ther. 1981; 30: 348–52.
43. Reimann IW, Diener U, Frölich JC. Indomethacin but not aspirin increases plasma lithium levels. Arch Gen Psychiatry. 1983; 40: 283–7.
44. Reimann I, Golbs E, Fischer C, Frölich JC. Influence of intravenous acetylsalicylic acid and sodium salicylate on human renal function and lithium clearance. Eur J Clin Pharmacol. 1985; 29: 435–41.
45. Flores AGA, Sharp GWG. Endogenous prostaglandins and osmotic water flow in the toad bladder. Am J Physiol. 1972; 223: 1392–7.
46. Frölich JC, Sweetman BJ, Carr K, Hollifield JW, Oates JA. Prostaglandin synthesis in rabbit renal medulla. Life Sci. 1975; 17: 1105–12.
47. Anderson RJ, Taber MS, Cronin RE, McDonald KM, Schrier RW. Effect of ß-adrenergic blockade and inhibitors of angiotensin II and prostaglandin on renal autoregulation. Am J Physiol. 1975; 229: 731–6.
48. Kramer HJ, Backer A, Hinzen S, Dusing R. Effects of inhibition of prostaglandin-synthesis on renal electrolyte excretion and concentrating ability in healthy man. Prostaglandins Med. 1978; 1: 341–9.
49. Urakabe S, Takamitsu Y, Shirai D et al. Effect of different prostaglandins on permeability of toad urinary bladder. Comp Biochem Physiol. 1975; 52:1–4.
50. Martinez F, Reyes JL. Prostaglandin receptors and hormonal action on water fluxes in cultured canine renal cells (MDCK line). J Physiol. 1984; 347: 533–43.
51. Grosse A, Cox JA, Malnoe A, deSousa RC. Evidence for a role of calmodulin in the hydroosmotic action of vasopressin in toad bladder. J Physiol. 1982; 19: 839–50.

52. Burch RM, Halushka PV. ^{45}Ca fluxes in isolated toad bladder epithelial cells: Effects of agents which alter water or sodium transport. J Pharmacol Exp Ther. 1983; 224: 108–17.
53. Bartelheimer HK, Senft G. Zur Lokalisation der tubulären Wirkung einiger antirheumatisch wirkender Substanzen. Arzneimittelforschung. 1968; 18: 567–70.
54. Culpepper RM, Andreoli TE. Interactions among prostaglandin E_2, antidiuretic hormone and cyclic adenosine monophosphate in modulating Cl$^-$ absorption in single mouse medullary thick ascending limbs of Henle. J Clin Invest. 1983; 71: 1588–601.
55. Bippi H, Frölich JC. Effects of acetylsalicylic acid and paracetamol alone and in combination on prostanoid synthesis in man. Br J Pharmacol. 1990; 29: 305–10.
56. Rosenkranz B, Fischer C, Frölich JC. Effects of salicylic and acetylsalicylic acid alone and in combination on platelet aggregation and prostanoid synthesis in man. Br J Clin Pharmacol. 1986; 21: 309–17.
57. Clive DM, Stoff JS. Renal syndromes associated with nonsteroidal antiinflammatory drugs. N Engl J Med. 1984; 310: 563–72.
58. Carmichael J, Shankel S. Effects of nonsteroidal anti-inflammatory drugs on prostaglandins and renal function. Am J Med. 1985; 78: 992–1000.
59. Flower RJ, Blackwell GJ. Anti-inflammatory steroids induce biosynthesis of a phospholipase A_2 inhibitor which prevents prostaglandin generation. Nature. 1979; 278: 456–9.
60. Naray-Fejes-Toth A, Fejes-Toth G, Fischer C, Frölich JC. Effect of dexamethasone on in vivo prostanoid production in the rabbit. J Clin Invest. 1984; 74: 120–3.
61. Rosenkranz B, Naray-Fejes-Toth A, Fejes-Toth G, Fischer C, Sawada M, Frölich JC. Dexamethasone effect on prostanoid formation in healthy man. Clin Sci. 1985; 68: 681–5.
62. Habenicht HJR, Goerig M, Grulich J et al. Human platelet derived growth factor stimulates prostaglandin synthesis by activation and rapid de novo synthesis of cyclooxygenase. J Clin Invest. 1985; 75: 1381–7.
63. Xie W, Chipman JG, Robertson DL, Erikson RL, Simmons D. Expression of a mitogen-responsive gene encoding prostaglandin synthase is regulated by mRNA splicing. Proc Natl Acad Sci USA. 1991; 88: 2692–5.
64. Kujubu DA, Fletcher BS, Varnum BC, Lim RW, Herschman HR. TIS10, a phorbol ester tumor promoter-inducible mRNA from Swiss 3T3 cells, encodes a novel prostaglandin synthase/cyclooxygenase homologue. J Biol Chem. 1991; 266: 12866–72.
65. Frölich JC. Prostaglandin endoperoxide synthetase isoenzymes: the clinical relevance of selective inhibition. Ann Rheum Dis. 1995; 54: 942–3.
66. Vane JR, Botting RM. New insights into the mode of action of anti-inflammatory drugs. Inflamm Res. 1995; 44: 1–9.
67. Smith WL, Bell TG. Immunohistochemical localization of the prostaglandin forming cyclooxygenase in renal cortex. Am J Physiol. 1978; 235: F451–7.
68. O'Neill GP, Ford-Hutchinson AW. Expression of mRNA for cyclooxygenase-1 and 2 in human tissues. FEBS Lett. 1993; 330: 156–60.
69. Harris RC, McKanna JA, Akai Y, Jacobson HR, Dubois RN, Breyer MD. Cyclooxygenase-2 is associated with the macula densa of rat kidney and increases with salt restriction. J Clin Invest. 1994; 94: 2504–10.
70. Pairet M, Churchill L, Engelhardt, G. Differential inhibition of cyclooxygenase 1 and 2 by NSAIDs. In: Bazan N, Botting J, Vane J (eds). New targets in inflammation: Inhibitors of COX-2 or adhesion molecules. Dordrecht: Kluwer Academic Publishers, 1996; 23–37.
71. Kujubu DA, Herschman HR. Dexamethasone inhibits mitogen induction of the TIS10 prostaglandin synthase/cyclooxygenase gene. J Biol Chem. 1992; 267: 7991–4.
72. Meade EA, Smith WL, DeWitt DL. Differential inhibition of prostaglandin endoperoxide synthase (cyclooxygenase) isozymes by aspirin and other non-steroidal antiinflammatory drugs. J Biol Chem. 1993; 268: 6610–14.
73. Klein T, Nüsing RM, Pfeilschifter J, Ullrich V. Selective inhibition of cyclooxygenase 2. Biochem Pharmacol. 1994; 48: 1605–10.
74. Mitchell JA, Akarasereenont P, Thiemermann C, Flower RJ, Vane JR. Selectivity of nonsteroidal antiinflammatory drugs as inhibitors of constitutive and inducible cyclooxygenase. Proc. Natl Acad Sci USA. 1994; 90: 11693–7.
75. Pairet M, Engelhardt G. Differential inhibition of COX-1 and COX-2 in vitro and

pharmacological profile in vivo of NSAIDs. In: Vane JR, Botting JH, Botting RM (eds). Improved non-steroid anti-inflammatory drugs: COX-2 enzyme inhibitors. Dordrecht: Kluwer Academic Publishers, and London: William Harvey Press, 1996: 103–19.

76. Engelhardt G, Bögel R, Schnitzer C, Utzmann R. Meloxicam: Influence on arachidonic acid metabolism. In vitro and in vivo findings (2 parts). Biochem Pharmacol. 1996; 51: 21–38.

77. Churchill L, Graham AG, Shuh CK, Pauletti D, Farina PR, Grob PM. Selective inhibition of human cyclo-oxygenase-2 by meloxicam. Inflammopharmacology. 1996; 4: 125–35.

78. Stichtenoth DO, Wagner B, Frölich JC. Effects of meloxicam and indomethacin on cyclooxygenase pathways in healthy volunteers. J Invest Med. 1997; 45: 44–9.

79. Bevis PJR, Bird HA, Lapham G. An open study to assess the safety and tolerability of meloxicam 15 mg in subjects with rheumatic disease and mild renal impairment. Brit J Rheumatol. 1996; 35 (suppl. 1): 56–60.

10 Aspirin-induced asthma and cyclooxygenases

R. J. GRYGLEWSKI

Bronchial asthma, irrespective of its specific triggers (allergens, cold, physical exercise or aspirin), is by and large an inflammatory disease. High plasma levels of immunoglobulin E (IgE), if present, indicate its atopic aetiology. Activated T lymphocytes (Th2) release various cytokines which promote recruitment, activation and secretion of mast cells, eosinophils and macrophages in the airways. Activation of these cells is associated with local release of pro-inflammatory, bronchoconstrictor or cytotoxic agents such as interleukins, proteases, superoxide anion (O_2^-), histamine, platelet activating factor (PAF) and a number of eicosanoids including sulphidopeptide-leukotrienes (LTC_4-E_4), leukotriene B_4(LTB_4), thromboxane A_2 (TXA_2), prostaglandins $F_{2\alpha}$ and D_2($PGF_{2\alpha}$ and PGD_2). These mediators contribute to an increase in vascular permeability, oedema, migration of leukocytes to tissues, epithelial shedding, fibroblast proliferation, bronchoconstriction, hyperreactivity of bronchi, rhinorrhea, cough and wheezing. Endogenous anti-inflammatory glucocorticoids, β adrenergic tone and the bronchodilator prostaglandin E_2 (PGE_2) counterbalance the pro-inflammatory cascade in the airways. Nitric oxide (NO) plays an ambiguous role in inflammatory response; however, in the lung it acts in opposition to pneumotoxic lipids (PAF, LTC_4-E_4, TXA_2), unless overproduction of NO, together with O_2^- yields toxic peroxynitrite ($ONOO^-$).

Although asthma is an inflammatory disease, asthmatic patients do not necessarily benefit from all types of anti-inflammatory drugs. Certainly, anti-inflammatory glucocorticoids applied either systemically or locally are the most powerful anti-asthmatic drugs. Selective β-adrenomimetics or stabilizers of mast cell and eosinophil membranes, such as cromoglycate disodium and nedocromil sodium, are also used in the therapy of asthma. However, for example, cyclosporine, an immunosuppressor of T lymphocytes, or antagonists of histamine H_1 receptors hold a modest position in anti-asthmatic therapy. PGE_2 inhalations are not used for the treatment of asthma since they produce cough and retrosternal pain. Aspirin and other non-steroidal anti-inflammatory drugs (NSAID) differentiate the adult population of asthmatic patients into three subgroups. Aspirin-tolerant asthma (ATA, 90% of patients), aspirin-induced asthma (AIA, 10% of patients) and aspirin-relieved asthma (ARA, 0.3% of patients). It is evident that only a few patients with asthma benefit from the treatment with aspirin: in most patients aspirin does not influence the course of the disease. In 10% of patients aspirin elicits acute asthmatic attacks, starting with wheezing, obstruction of airflow, sometimes accompanied by rhinorrhea, urticaria, angioedema, coronary vasospasm and other vascular disturbances. This paradox of AIA patients will be the subject of this chapter.

EARLY STUDIES

Experimental models of AIA do not exist, and hence until now studies on AIA have been confined to patients. Typical clinical methods consist of a challenge with aspirin (ASA) or soluble lysyl aspirin (LASA) at doses ranging from 0.5 to 300 mg given orally, intravenously, transdermally, intranasally, by inhalation or by intrabronchial instillation. The resultant bronchospasm is measured as a decrease in peak expiratory flow (PEF) or in forced expiratory volume during 1 second (FEV_1), or maximum expiratory flow (MEF). Biological samples for assay consist of blood, airway biopsies, nasal polyps, nasal lavage, bronchoalveolar lavage (BAL) or urine.

Reports on adverse reactions to aspirin in asthmatic patients appeared soon after it was marketed at the turn of the century. In these 'aspirin-sensitive' asthmatics, treatment with gradually increasing doses of aspirin could evoke tolerance to its harmful effects. Reports on co-existence of idiosyncrasy to a yellow food dye, tartrazine, supported an obvious assumption that 'aspirin-sensitive' asthma was one more example of allergy to chemicals. In the mid seventies immunological studies excluded allergy as a cause of AIA[1], later the myth of an association between aspirin and tartrazine as inducers of AIA was disproved[2], and thus intolerance to aspirin is established as a phenomenon which is not dependent on an allergic reaction.

THE COX THEORY

Inspired by John Vane's discovery on the mechanism of action of aspirin[3], we decided to examine whether this mechanism might explain the untoward reactions to aspirin in AIA patients. Indeed, in 1975 we reported that AIA patients would react with bronchospasm not only to a challenge with aspirin, but also to a challenge with four other NSAIDs with chemical structures distinct from aspirin (indomethacin, flufenamate, mefenamate and phenylbutazone)[1]. A common feature of these four NSAIDs and aspirin was their inhibitory action on cyclooxygenase (COX-1) in bovine seminal vesicle microsomes in vitro. Four other analgesics, including salicylamide, which had no effect on activity of COX in vitro could be safely ingested by AIA patients producing no harmful effects. Moreover, we found a rough correlation between in vitro COX inhibitory potencies of NSAID (corrected for their albumin-binding capacities) and their clinical efficacies to evoke bronchospasm in AIA patients. In each of 11 AIA patients, the severity of adverse reactions to the NSAID studied was intensified by increasing its dosage, thus differing from a typical allergenic response. We therefore proposed that the pathogenesis of AIA is closely related to the inhibition of prostanoid biosynthesis in the airways. Our original observation was reinforced in our next studies[4,5]. We extended the list of COX inhibitors inducing AIA with ibuprofen, fenoprofen and diclofenac while other authors added naproxen and ketoprofen. Statistical analysis in eighteen AIA patients proved that each of them had their own individual hallmark of the 'sensitivity' to aspirin. In each patient the threshold effective dose of aspirin enabled one to predict the range of sensitivity to the other COX inhibitors[4,5]. Thus the theory was formulated that in AIA patients adverse reactions to aspirin (bronchospasm, rhinorrhoea, angioedema, urticaria) are triggered by inhibition of COX and not by allergy to salicylates. Strong support for the COX theory is the fact that AIA patients in whom tolerance to aspirin was induced also became insensitive to the deleterious action of other COX inhibitors such as diclofenac or indomethacin[6].

What is the difference between cyclooxygenases in airways of patients belonging to ATA, ARA and AIA subtypes of asthma? This essential question still remains unanswered. One possibility is that in AIA patients COX in certain cellular compartments (e.g. in eosinophils) is more accessible to NSAID than in others[5]. The second possibility is that chronic viral infection evokes transcriptional aberrations in constructing COX in the airways of AIA patients. Another option is that cytotoxic lymphocytes, when killing virus-affected cells, release toxins which then precipitate asthmatic attacks[7]. This 'viral hypothesis' of AIA is supported by clinical evidence (AIA frequently begins with a respiratory infection), pharmacological evidence (acyclovir attenuates AIA) and immunological evidence (a rise in IgG4 in AIA patients points to a chronic response to a viral antigen). It is still a matter of dispute as to whether a defect of COX in AIA patients is restricted to their airways or is a generalized phenomenon.

THE ROLE OF CORTICOIDS IN AIA

In AIA patients pretreatment with corticoids reduces the adverse reactions to a challenge with aspirin. This protective action of corticoids is taken for granted because corticoids are known to protect against bronchospasm in any type of asthma. Possible mechanisms are the inhibitory action of corticoids on release of interleukin-2 from T cells or on release of LTC_4-E_4 and PGD_2 from eosinophils and mast cells, possibly by preventing induction of the relevant generating enzymes. However in one study, three out of 31 AIA patients injected with hydrocortisone hemisuccinate (50–300 mg i.v.) developed an instant bronchospasm (a drop in $FEV_1 > 20\%$)[8]. Similarly, the extensive Japanese epidemiological study in 850 asthmatic patients (ATA patients, 88% and AIA patients, 12% of the cohort) revealed six AIA patients who did not tolerate intravenous hydrocortisone. None of the ATA patients showed an adverse reaction to corticoids[9]. The reason for a dramatic obstruction of airways by hydrocortisone in 6–10% of AIA patients is unknown, but one has to keep in mind that corticoids exert their action on arachidonate metabolism not only through a delayed transcriptional mechanism on inducible enzymes, but also through an instantaneous mechanism by preventing the mobilization of the substrate for COX-1 from phospholipids[10]. It may well be that in the fraction of AIA patients who do not tolerate hydrocortisone, its instant inhibitory action on the generation of PGE_2 prevails over its retarded inhibitory influence on the biosynthesis of deleterious prostanoids and sulphidopeptide leukotrienes, as is the case with NSAID (see below).

THE PGE$_2$ HYPOTHESIS

In the first three papers in which we associated NSAID-induced bronchospasm in AIA patients with COX inhibition[1,4,5] we also formulated a hypothesis for the pathomechanism of AIA. This hypothesis has been continuously revised but its basic premise is unchanged. The fact that COX-inhibitors bring about bronchospasm in a subpopulation of asthmatic patients suggests that PGE_2 is the primary cause of the phenomenon simply because AIA patients are more likely to suffer from inhibition of the biosynthesis of cytoprotective and bronchodilator PGE_2 than from removal of the pro-inflammatory and bronchoconstrictor $PGF_{2\alpha}$, PGD_2 or TXA_2. PGI_2 is obviously not involved because it does not protect AIA patients from ASA-induced asthmatic attacks. Arising from the PGE_2 hypothesis various conceptions developed on differences in response to NSAID between AIA and ATA patients. For instance, in contrast with ATA patients, AIA patients are supposed to rely more on PGE_2 than on β-adrenergic tone in defending their lungs against noxious stimuli[1,5]. Indeed, inhaled PGE_2 is highly effective in preventing AIA[11] and its action is stronger than that of salbutamol if both drugs are compared at equimolar concentrations[12]. Other evidence stems from the finding that slices of nasal polyps from AIA patients when compared with those from non-asthmatic patients were more susceptible to the inhibitory action of aspirin on the generation of PGE_2[5]. Interestingly, this difference disappeared when, instead of slices, homogenates of polyps were used, as if the 'hypersensitivity' to aspirin in AIA patients was associated with a peculiarity in cell structure rather than with an anomaly in the enzyme itself. However, the strongest evidence for a selective inhibition of the biosynthesis of PGE_2 by aspirin in AIA patients comes from the recent paper by Szczeklik and his colleagues[13]. AIA and ATA patients were challenged intrabronchially with LASA. Apart from FEV_1 the authors measured the number of cells and the concentrations of a broad range of eicosanoids in BAL fluid. In ATA patients aspirin at doses which decreased FEV_1 by more than 20% also produced a uniform inhibition of prostanoid levels in BAL. In contrast with ATA patients, in those with AIA aspirin lowered only PGE_2 and TXA_2 levels, not those of other prostanoids. Perhaps NSAID-evoked selective deficiency in pulmonary PGE_2 enhances the effects of the bronchoconstrictor prostanoids, $PGF_{2\alpha}$ or PGD_2. TXA_2 cannot be involved because its generation in BAL of AIA patients is inhibited by aspirin along with suppression of PGE_2 production[13]; moreover, inhibition of TXA_2 synthase by OKY-046, though lowering plasma TXB_2 levels and causing an increase in the level of 6-keto-$PGF_{1\alpha}$, does not affect bronchopulmonary function in AIA patients[14]. Obviously, prostacyclin and thromboxane do not participate in the adverse reactions to NSAID in AIA patients.

THE $PGF_{2\alpha}$ AND PGD_2 HYPOTHESIS

$PGF_{2\alpha}$ and PGD_2 are bronchoconstrictors in human airways. Perhaps the airways of AIA patients are unduly sensitive to $PGF_{2\alpha}$ or PGD_2, since during challenge with aspirin their biosynthesis is not impaired yet PGE_2 disappears from BAL[13]. There is little support for the involvement of $PGF_{2\alpha}$. AIA patients do not seem to be more sensitive to inhaled $PGF_{2\alpha}$, or indeed to histamine, than ATA patients, though NSAID more effectively displaces $PGF_{2\alpha}$ from serum proteins of AIA patients as compared to ATA patients[15], thus leaving more of the unbound bronchoconstrictor available. Apart from histamine, mast cells are known to release PGD_2. Bronchial biopsies from

AIA patients show infiltration with mast cells and challenge with aspirin is associated with an increase in serum levels of tryptase and histamine[16], pointing to activation of mast cells. Similarly, aspirin-challenge in AIA, but not in ATA, patients dose-dependently increased urinary excretion of $9\alpha,11\beta$-PGF_2, a stable metabolite of PGD_2, and this was correlated with the decrease in bronchopulmonary function of AIA patients[17]. The involvement of PGD_2 in AIA attacks was also indicated by an immunochemical study[18] on numbers of inflammatory cells in the bronchial mucosa of AIA patients following intrabronchial challenge with aspirin. A decrease in both absolute mast cell numbers staining with mastocyte tryptase (mAb AA1), and the percentage of mast cells co-immunostaining with pAb LOX-5 may represent degranulation of these cells. It is likely that activated mast cells also release PGD_2 along with histamine and leukotrienes.

THE LEUKOTRIENE HYPOTHESIS

In the same study[18] biopsies of bronchial mucosa from AIA patients also contained an increased number of total (mAb MBK13) and activated (mAb EG2) eosinophils. Nasal polyps (which are found in a half of AIA patients) were also rich in activated eosinophils[19]. Accumulation of activated mast cells and eosinophils in the airways of AIA patients surpasses that in ATA patients and it is not associated with an increased infiltration with neutrophils, macrophages and lymphocytes[18,19]. Activated mast cells and eosinophils are known to generate, or to initiate the generation of, sulphidopeptide leukotrienes (LTC_4-LTE_4). Originally, a role of LTC_4-LTE_4 in pathogenesis of AIA was automatically assumed, since a blockade of COX by NSAID was supposed to redirect the non-consumed pool of arachidonate to the 5-lipoxygenase(LOX) pathway. It appears that this 'shunt hypothesis' is no longer satisfactory[20] even though during a challenge with aspirin of AIA patients, the selective inhibition of PGE_2 generation is accompanied by a dramatic increase in LTC_4-LTE_4 levels in their BAL fluid[13]. A link between these two observations might be as follows. In AIA patients biosynthesis of LTs by inflammatory cells in bronchial mucosa (mast cells and eosinophils) is kept at bay owing to the brake imposed by PGE_2. Its removal by NSAID causes a dramatic increase in the biosynthesis of LTs. Alternatively, in AIA patients, perhaps PGE_2 is critically required to blunt the bronchoconstrictor and proinflammatory actions of LTC_4-E_4. The study of Arm et al.[21] favours the latter explanation. In AIA patients inhaled LTE_4 was 1870 times more potent as a bronchoconstrictor than histamine. In ATA patients this ratio was only 145. After desensitization to aspirin of AIA patients, their ratio of reactivity to LTE_4/histamine fell from 1870 to 58. It is thus apparent that hypersensitivity to the bronchoconstrictor action of LTE_4 is associated with the active AIA syndrome and disappears when patients are temporarily desensitized to aspirin. Still another possibility is that formation of lipoxin A_4 (LXA_4) may contribute to AIA attacks[22].

Clinical studies with antileukotriene agents hold promise to add LT-receptor antagonists and LT synthesis inhibitors to the existing classes of anti-asthmatic drugs. Though these studies have already helped to elucidate some aspects of pathophysiology of bronchial asthma[23], it is difficult to distinguish LT-related asthmas from other types. So far it seems that most types of asthma may benefit from intervention with anti-leukotriene agents. It is likely, however, that such therapy will be preferentially effective in AIA patients[24].

Another interesting feature of the leukotriene hypothesis emerges from observations that AIA patients may also suffer from Prinzmetal variant angina[25], Churg-Strauss syndrome (granulomatous angiitis)[26], autoimmune vasculiitis[27], isolated periorbital angioedema[28] or other vascular disorders. The detrimental effects of transcellular transfer of LTA_4 from activated leukocytes to the effector cells which contain LTC_4 synthase were described in cardiovascular system[29]. The coincidence of bronchial and vascular harmful effects of COX-inhibitors in AIA patients may be explained by mobilization of activated eosinophils and mast cells, followed by a transcellular transportation of LTA_4 from these inflammatory cells to bronchial or vascular walls, which then generate LTC_4-E_4. These lipids are injurious in statu nascendi within either bronchial or arterial walls.

ASPIRIN-RELIEVED ASTHMA

The mechanism of aspirin-relieved asthma (ARA) remains a mystery. ARA is also relieved by other COX inhibitors such as mefenamate or ketoprofen, but most interestingly, asthma is precipitated in ARA patients by 5-LOX inhibitors such as AA 861[30].

CONCLUSIONS

Inhibition of COX by NSAID in the airways plays a crucial role in the adverse reactions to aspirin and to other NSAID in AIA patients. An anomaly in COX, in PG isomerases or in cellular accessibility of COX to NSAID appears to be involved but its nature remains unknown. The significance of COX-1/COX-2 inhibitory ratio of NSAID for the cause of bronchospasm in AIA patients is under study. A selective removal of PGE_2 by NSAID from the airways of AIA patients seems to be crucial. The PGE_2 deficiency uncovers the bronchoconstrictor activity of its positional isomer PGD_2 released from activated mast cells. Weakening of PGE_2-mediated braking mechanisms also allows leukocytes, mainly eosinophils, to generate pneumotoxic sulphidopeptide leukotrienes (LTC_4-E_4). A similar transcellular mechanism of synthesis of LTC_4-E_4 in the vascular system might be responsible for the coexisting vascular disorders in AIA patients (Figure 1).

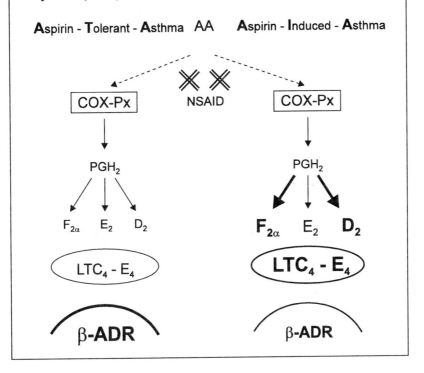

Figure 1. A hypothesis for the mechanism of AIA. Cyclooxygenase (COX), within the prostaglandin H synthase complex (COX-Px), responds differently to inhibition by non-steroidal antiinflammatory drugs (NSAID) in the airways of patients with aspirin-tolerant asthma (ATA) compared with patients with aspirin-induced-asthma (AIA). In ATA patients NSAIDs suppress equally the generation of all prostaglandins, and the pulmonary production of sulphidopeptide leukotrienes (LTC₄-E₄) is not affected. Consequently, NSAIDs do not change a balance between pro-asthmatic LTC₄-E₄, PGD₂, PGF₂, and anti-asthmatic PGE₂. Further, in airways of ATA patients β-adrenergic tone is sufficient to maintain bronchiolar dilation even during PGE₂ deficiency. In AIA patients NSAIDs selectively inhibit the generation of PGE₂[13,17], giving way for the bronchoconstrictor and proinflammatory actions of PGD₂ and PGF₂ released from mast cells and eosinophils[18]. In addition, in AIA patients selective PGE₂ deficiency is responsible for the over-production of LTC₄-E₄ in the airways[13,20]

References

1. Szczeklik A, Gryglewski RJ, Czerniawska-Mysik G. Relationship of inhibition of prostaglandin biosynthesis by analgesics to asthma attacks in aspirin-sensitive patients. Br Med J. 1975; 1: 67–9.
2. Virchow C, Szczeklik A, Bianco S et al. Intolerance to tartrazine in aspirin-induced asthma: results of a multicenter study. Respiration. 1988; 53: 20–33.
3. Vane JR. Inhibition of prostaglandin biosynthesis as the mechanism of action of aspirin-like drugs. Nature New Biol. 1971; 23: 232–5.

4. Szczeklik A, Gryglewski RJ, Czerniawska-Mysik G, Żmuda A. Aspirin-induced asthma. J Allergy Clin Immunol. 1976; 58: 10–18.

5. Gryglewski RJ, Szczeklik A, Niżankowska E. Aspirin-sensitive asthma: Its relationship to inhibition of prostaglandin biosynthesis. In: Berti F, Samuelsson B, Velo JP (eds). Prostaglandins and Thromboxanes. New York: Plenum Press, 1977: 191–203.

6. Szmidt M, Grzelewska-Rzymowska I, Rozneicki J. Tolerance to aspirin in aspirin-sensitive asthmatics. Methods of inducing the tolerance state and its influence on the course of asthma and rhinosinusitis. J Invest Allergol Clin Immunol. 1993; 3: 156–9.

7. Szczeklik A. Aspirin-induced asthma as a viral disease. Clin Allergy. 1988; 8: 15–20.

8. Szczeklik A, Niżankowska E, Czerniakwska-Mysik G, Sêk S. Hydrocortisone and airflow impairment in aspirin-induced asthma. J Allergy Clin Immunol. 1985; 6: 530–6.

9. Enomoto T, Okada T, Ichihashi K et al. Questionnaire to 850 asthmatics on hypersensitivity to non-steroidal anti-inflammatory drugs and hypersensitivity to steroids. Arerugi. 1995; 44: 534–9.

10. Gryglewski RJ, Panczenko B, Korbut R, Grodzińska L, Ocetkiewicz A. Corticosteroids inhibit prostaglandin release from perfused mesenteric blood vessels of rabbit and from perfused lungs of sensitized guinea pig. Prostaglandins. 1975; 10: 343–56.

11. Sestini P, Armetti L, Gambaro G et al. Inhaled PGE_2 prevents aspirin-induced bronchoconstriction and urinary LTE_4 excretion in aspirin-sensitive asthma. Am J Resp Crit Care Med. 1996; 153: 572–5.

12. Szczeklik A, Mastalerz L, Niżankowska E, Cmiel A. Protective and bronchodilaton effects of prostaglandin E and salbutamol in aspirin-induced asthma. Am J Resp Crit Care Med. 1996; 153: 567–71.

13. Szczeklik A, Sladek K, Dworski R et al. Bronchial aspirin challenge causes specific eicosanoid response in aspirin-sensitive asthmatics. Am J Resp Crit Care Med. 1996; 154: 1608–14.

14. Szczeklik A, Niżankowska E, Spławiński J, Dworski R, Gajewski P, Spławińska B. Effects of inhibition of thromboxane A_2 synthesis in aspirin-induced asthma. J Allergy Clin Immunol. 1987; 80: 839–43.

15. Williams WR, Pawłowicz A, Davies BH. Aspirin-sensitive asthma: significance of the cyclooxygenase-inhibiting and protein-binding properties of analgesic drugs. Int Arch Allergy Appl Immunol. 1991; 95: 303–8.

16. Lane SJ, Lee TH. Mast cell effector mechanisms. J Allergy Clin Immunol. 1996; 98: S67–S71.

17. O'Sullivan S, Dahlen B, Dahlen SE, Kumlin M. Increased urinary excretion of the prostaglandin D-2 metabolite 9 alpha, 11 beta-prostaglandin F-2 after aspirin challenge supports mast cell activation in aspirin-induced airway obstruction. J Allergy Clin Immunol. 1996; 98: 421–32.

18. Nasser S, Christie PE, Pfister R et al. Effect of endobronchial aspirin challenge on inflammatory cells in bronchial biopsy samples from aspirin-sensitive asthmatic subjects. Thorax. 1996; 51: 64–70.

19. Yoshimi R, Takamura H, Takasaki K, Tsurumoto H, Kumagami H. Immunohistological study of eosinophilic infiltration of nasal polyps in aspirin-induced asthma. Nippon Jibiinkoka Gakkai Kaiho. 1993; 96: 1922–5.

20. Knapp HR, Sladek K, Fitzgerald GA. Increased excretion of leukotriene E_4 during aspirin-induced asthma. J Lab Clin Med. 1992; 119: 48–51.

21. Arm JP, O'Hickey SP, Spur BW, Lee TH. Airway responsiveness to histamine and leukotriene E_4 in subjects with aspirin-induced asthma. Am Rev Resp Dis. 1989; 140: 148–53.

22. Levy BD, Bertram S, Tai HH et al. Agonist-induced lipoxin A_4 generation: detection by a novel lipoxin A_4-ELISA. Lipids. 1993; 28: 1047–53.

23. Smith LJ. Leukotrienes in asthma. The potential therapeutic role of antileukotriene agents. Arch Intern Med. 1996; 156: 2181–9.

24. Ind PW. Anti-leukotriene intervention: Is there adequate information for clinical use in asthma? Resp Med. 1996; 90: 575–86.

25. Habbab MA, Szwed SA, Haft JI. Is coronary arterial spasm part of the aspirin-induced asthma syndrome? Chest. 1986; 90: 141–3.

26. Suzuki N, Arai Y, Miyamoto Y, Isokane N, Fukushima N, Sano Y. Acute myocardial injury

and repeated angina pectoris-like attacks in a young patient with Churg-Strauss syndrome. Nippon Kyobu Shikkan Gakkai Zasshi. 1991; 29: 1630–7.

27. Szczeklik A, Musiał J, Dyczek A, Bartosik A, Milewski M. Autoimmune vasculitis preceding aspirin-induced asthma. Int Arch Allergy Immunol. 1995: 106: 92–4.

28. Quiralte J, Blanco C, Castillo R, Delgado J, Carrillo T. Intolerance to nonsteroidal antiinflammatory drugs: Results of controlled drug challenges in 98 patients. J Allergy Clin Immunol. 1996; 98: 678–85.

29. Sala A, Aliev GM, Rossoni G et al. Morphological and functional changes of coronary vasculature caused by transcellular biosynthesis of sulfidopeptide leukotrienes in isolated heart of rabbit. Blood. 1996; 87: 1824–32.

30. Imokawa S, Sato A, Taniguchi M, Toyoshima M, Hayakawa H, Chida K. Lipoxygenase inhibitor-provoked acute asthma in a patient with asthma relieved by aspirin. Ann Allergy Asthma Immunol. 1995; 75: 112–14.

11 New classification of aspirin-like drugs

H. FENNER

The discovery of two distinct isoforms of cyclooxygenase (COX) has promoted a better understanding of the anti-inflammatory and toxicity profiles of non-steroidal anti-inflammatory drugs (NSAIDs). Prostanoids that are derived from the COX-1 pathway regulate platelet aggregation via thromboxane A_2 (TXA_2), the function and integrity of the gut mucosa, and kidney function via prostaglandin E_2 (PGE_2) and prostacyclin. COX-2 is expressed in various cell types, including monocytes, fibroblasts and synovial cells, in response to inflammatory stimuli (e.g. cytokines and endotoxin). Consequently, COX-1 inhibition by NSAIDs is associated with gastrointestinal and renal toxicity, whereas, COX-2 inhibition limits the formation of pro-inflammatory and nociceptive prostanoids at the site of the inflammatory response.

NSAIDs vary considerably in terms of their selectivity for COX-2 relative to COX-1. The relative efficacy of a drug may be considered to be due to synovial COX-2 inhibitory activity, whereas the relative toxicity may be considered to be due to systemic COX-1 inhibitory activity. Since NSAIDs at anti-inflammatory dosages can be considered equipotent, synovial COX-2 activity must be inhibited to a similar extent. Differences in the toxicity of NSAIDs must therefore be related to systemic COX-1 inhibition in the cells that express this isoform (i.e. the gastrointestinal mucosa and renal tissue). Experimental data on systemic inhibition of COX-1 relative to the synovial inhibition of COX-2 may prove to be useful in predicting the risk of gastrointestinal toxicity with these drugs and could provide a rationale for the classification of NSAIDs according to their benefit/risk ratio. This should offer a more clinically meaningful classification than previous approaches, which are based solely on chemical or pharmacological criteria.

MODELS FOR THE EVALUATION OF COX-1 AND COX-2 INHIBITORY ACTIVITY

Various experimental models have been developed to study the differential inhibitory activity of NSAIDs on the COX-2/COX-1 isoforms. These include different cell systems using free enzymes, human recombinant enzymes, purified enzymes and enzymes from non-human sources. The selectivity of NSAIDs for the COX-1 and COX-2 isoforms has been assessed from these systems by calculating the concentration of a drug causing 50% inhibition (IC_{50}) of COX-1 and COX-2, and expressing the two values as a ratio (COX-2/COX-1). The lower the ratio, the more potently the drug inhibits COX-2 relative to COX-1. However, important differences in experimental conditions between the models have resulted in variations in IC_{50}

measurements between the different assay systems. For instance, as NSAIDs are highly protein-bound in the blood, the active concentration of drug is strongly influenced by the protein concentration in the assay medium. Many cell-free systems use artificially high concentrations of arachidonate substrate compared with intact cell systems, which might influence the susceptibility of COX-1 and COX-2 to NSAIDs. The inhibition of COX activity by some NSAIDs is time dependent[1] and, therefore, different incubation times produce different results. Such inter- and intra-assay variability results in large differences in the COX-2/COX-1 ratio of individual NSAIDs, raising doubts over the clinical significance of the models used and the COX-2/COX-1 ratios obtained.

More recently, human whole blood assays have been used to investigate the differential inhibition of the COX isoforms. In vitro systems use whole blood taken from human donors to test the inhibitory activity on COX-1 and COX-2[1-7]. Ex vivo models use blood samples from healthy subjects or patients who have taken NSAIDs in therapeutic dosages over a period of several days[8,9]. The latter has the benefit of allowing the effects of NSAIDs to be studied in the steady-state, more accurately reflecting their therapeutic activity. Data obtained from human whole blood assays are more clinically relevant with respect to COX-1 and COX-2 inhibition, as they reflect the important pharmacokinetic and pharmacodynamic factors affecting the drug's activity. Since only a fraction of the NSAID is able to enter the platelet or monocyte and interact with the active site of the COX enzymes in the endoplasmic reticulum, the model takes into account the role of protein-binding and the physico-chemical factors defining the rate and extent of transmembrane transport and intracellular trapping.

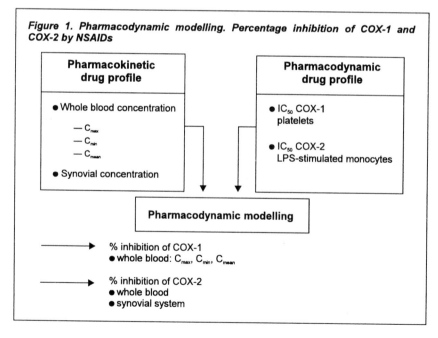

Figure 1. Pharmacodynamic modelling. Percentage inhibition of COX-1 and COX-2 by NSAIDs

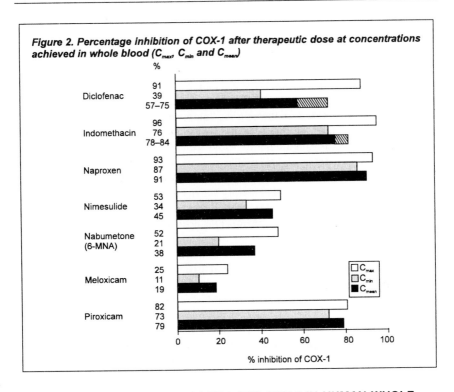

Figure 2. Percentage inhibition of COX-1 after therapeutic dose at concentrations achieved in whole blood (C_{max}, C_{min} and C_{mean})

DIFFERENTIAL INHIBITION OF COX-1 AND COX-2 IN HUMAN WHOLE BLOOD ASSAYS

The selectivity of COX-1 and COX-2 inhibition by NSAIDs has been studied by several groups using in vitro human whole blood assays. Patrignani et al.[2] measured TXB_2 levels as a reflection of platelet COX-1 activity, and used lipopolysaccharide (LPS)-stimulated monocytes as a marker of COX-2 activity. Brideau et al.[3] measured PGE_2 levels in LPS-stimulated human whole blood and TXB_2 levels after blood coagulation as biochemical markers of COX-2 and COX-1 activity, respectively. Both Glaser et al.[1] and Young et al.[4] described the COX selectivity of a range of NSAIDs, using the release of TXB_2 from platelets in whole blood from healthy male donors as a measure of COX-1 activity, and TXB_2 release from LPS-stimulated whole blood (principally from monocytes) as a COX-2 specific assay. These studies investigated a variety of standard NSAIDs, and provided IC_{50} data for both COX-1 and COX-2 isoforms. Also available are plasma drug concentrations at certain timepoints after the administration of therapeutic dosages of various NSAIDs, including indomethacin[10], diclofenac[11,12], piroxicam[13], meloxicam[14], naproxen[15], nimesulide[16] and nabumetone[17]. The relationship between drug concentration at equipotent anti-inflammatory dosages and COX-1 inhibitory activity as measured in the human whole blood assay can be determined using pharmacodynamic modelling[18] (Figure 1). The modelling uses a drug's pharmacokinetic profile (whole blood and synovial drug concentrations) and pharmacodynamic profile (IC_{50} COX-1 in platelets; IC_{50} COX-2 in LPS-stimulated monocytes) to derive the percentage inhibition of COX-1 in whole blood (C_{max}, C_{min}, C_{mean}) and the percentage inhibition of COX-2 (in whole blood and in the synovial system).

At mean whole blood drug levels corresponding to levels attained after therapeutic doses, all of the NSAIDs analysed for this relationship, except nabumetone, were potent inhibitors of COX-2, confirming the equipotency of their anti-inflammatory activity. In contrast, there was much greater variability of COX-1 inhibition, ranging from <20% with meloxicam 7.5 mg to >90% with naproxen 500 mg bid (Table 1). Nabumetone had a more favourable profile for COX-1 inhibition (38% at steady state after 1000 mg) but also has low COX-2 inhibitory activity (40%), reflecting the drug's good tolerability but low anti-inflammatory activity at such dosages.

It is important to examine COX-1 inhibitory activity over the range of drug concentrations attained following therapeutic doses of NSAIDs. Comparison of COX-1 inhibitory activity at minimum, mean and maximum blood drug levels achieved after therapeutic doses demonstrates marked differences between NSAIDs (Figure 2). Around three hours after the administration of diclofenac 50 mg, COX-1 was inhibited by 91% at maximum plasma drug levels; however, 5 hours later this was reduced to 39%. The diclofenac 100 mg controlled release formulation exerted a mean

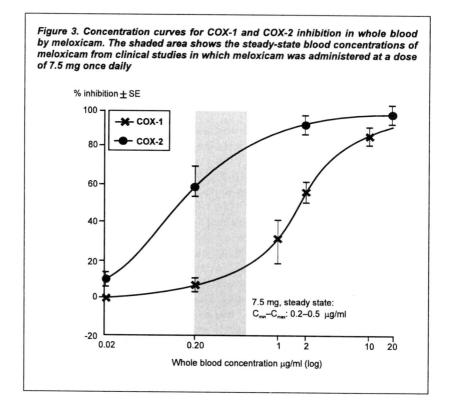

Figure 3. Concentration curves for COX-1 and COX-2 inhibition in whole blood by meloxicam. The shaded area shows the steady-state blood concentrations of meloxicam from clinical studies in which meloxicam was administered at a dose of 7.5 mg once daily

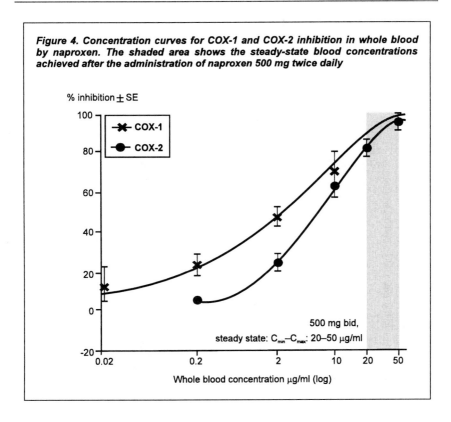

Figure 4. Concentration curves for COX-1 and COX-2 inhibition in whole blood by naproxen. The shaded area shows the steady-state blood concentrations achieved after the administration of naproxen 500 mg twice daily

inhibition of between 57% and 75%. By comparison, naproxen had more or less equal inhibitory effects on COX-1 over a 24 hour dosing interval; COX-1 was almost completely inhibited (93%) at maximum plasma levels after a 500 mg dose and was still inhibited by 87% before the next dose was administered 12 hours later.

Patrono's group[2,5] and Pairet et al.[6,7] used the human whole blood assay in vitro to investigate the inhibitory activity of several NSAIDs, including the new drug meloxicam, on the COX isoforms. TXB_2 levels were measured as a reflection of platelet COX-1 activity, while PGE_2 formation in LPS-stimulated monocytes was taken as a marker of COX-2 activity. Concentration–response relationships determined for meloxicam and naproxen are presented in Figures 3 and 4, respectively. At whole blood drug concentrations of between 0.2 and 0.5 µg/ml, corresponding to plasma levels attained after therapeutic doses of meloxicam (7.5 mg), COX-1 activity was inhibited by around 10% and COX-2 activity was inhibited by around 80%. By comparison, therapeutic dosages of naproxen (500 mg twice daily) induced almost complete inhibition of COX-1 (90%) and COX-2 (85%) activity. These data clearly show that meloxicam inhibits COX-2 more potently than COX-1 and are consistent with the lack of effect of meloxicam on COX-1 mediated TXA_2 formation in volunteers[8].

Table 1. Whole blood concentrations (C_{max}, C_{min}, C_{mean}) and COX-1 inhibition of various NSAIDs

NSAID	IC_{50} COX-1 (µg/ml)	NSAID dose	Whole blood concentration (µg/ml) and COX-1 inhibition (%)						Reference	
			C_{max} [hours]	COX-1 inhibition	C_{min} [hours]	COX-1 inhibition	C_{mean} [hours]	COX-1 inhibition	IC_{50}	Kinetics
Diclofenac	0.045	50 mg tid	0.44 [3]	91	0.033 [8]	39			3	11
		100 mg SR					0.06–0.12 [4–8]	57–73		12
Indomethacin	0.061	50 mg	1.6 [1]	96	0.19 [9]	76	0.22–0.33 [3–7]	78–84	7	10
Naproxen	3.9	500 mg bid day 7	49 [2]	93	23 [12]	86	35	90	2–5	15
Nimesulide	2.7	2×100 mg	3.0 [3]	53	1.4 [12]	34	2.2	45	2–5	16
Nabumetone (6-MNA)	66	1 g/day	72	52	23 [24]	21	41	38	2–5	17
Meloxicam	1.7	7.5 mg	0.58 [5]	25	0.2 [24]	11	0.4	19	2–5	14
Piroxicam	0.95	20 mg	4.4 [3]	82	2.5 [24]	73	3.5	79	2–5	13

It may be concluded that COX-1 inhibitory activity at therapeutic drug concentrations differs greatly between NSAIDs. Theoretically a range of NSAIDs can be identified, from aspirin, which has mainly COX-1 inhibitory effects, to drugs such as meloxicam which preferentially inhibit COX-2. It is clear that those NSAIDs that are selective towards COX-2 have clinically significant advantages over conventional non-selective drugs in terms of gastrointestinal and renal toxicity profiles at anti-inflammatory dosages. The improved tolerability profile of meloxicam over standard NSAIDs has been demonstrated in large comparative clinical trials[19].

CONCLUSIONS

The human whole blood assay provides a meaningful model for the determination of the differential inhibition of COX-2 relative to COX-1, taking into account the pharmacokinetic and physicochemical factors affecting the distribution of NSAIDs. The model can be used as a clinically relevant source of information for classifying NSAIDs according to their COX-2 inhibition: COX-1 inhibition ratio. This ratio reflects major differences between NSAIDs with respect to COX-1 inhibition at doses exerting equipotent COX-2 inhibitory, and hence, anti-inflammatory, activity in patients.

Differential COX-2/COX-1 inhibition, as determined using a meaningful model, presents a rationale for classifying NSAIDs by ranking them according to their ratio: synovial COX-2 (%) inhibition/systemic COX-1 (%) inhibition. In contrast to previous approaches, which classify NSAIDs by chemical or pharmacological criteria, this classification expresses the differences in gastrointestinal toxicity demonstrated in clinical and pharmaco-epidemiological studies.

References

1. Glaser KB. Cyclooxygenase selectivity and NSAIDs: Cyclooxygenase-2 selectivity of etodolac (Lodine). Inflammopharmacology. 1995; 3: 335–45.
2. Patrignani P, Panara MR, Greco A et al. Biochemical and pharmacological characterization of the cyclooxygenase activity of human blood prostaglandin endoperoxide synthases. J Pharmacol Exp Ther. 1994; 271: 1705–12.
3. Brideau C, Kargman S, Liu S et al. A human whole blood assay for clinical evaluation of biochemical efficacy of cyclooyxgenase inhibitors. Inflamm Res. 1996; 45: 68–74.
4. Young JM, Panah S, Satchawatcharaphong C, Cheung PS. Human whole blood assays for inhibition of prostaglandin G/H synthases-1 and -2 using A23187 and lipopolysaccharide stimulation of thromboxane B2 production. Inflamm Res. 1996; 45: 246–53.
5. Patrignani P, Panara MR, Santini G et al. Differential inhibition of the cyclooxygenase activity of prostaglandin endoperoxide synthase isozymes in vitro and ex vivo in man. 10th Int Conf on Prostaglandins and Related Compounds, Vienna, Sep 1996. Prostaglandins Leukot Essent Fatty Acids. 1996; 55 (Suppl 1): 98.
6. Pairet M, Engelhardt G. Differential inhibition of COX-1 and COX-2 in vitro and pharmacokinetic profile in vivo of NSAIDs. In: Vane J, Botting J, Botting R (eds). Improved Non-steroid Anti-inflammatory Drugs – COX-2 Enzyme Inhibitors. Dordrecht: Kluwer Academic Publishers, 1996: 103–19.
7. Pairet M. Differential inhibition of COX-1/COX-2 by NSAIDs. William Harvey Research Conference on Selective COX-2 Inhibitors: Pharmacology, Clinical Effects and Therapeutic Potential; March 1997; Cannes, France.

8. Stichtenoth DO, Wagner B, Frölich JC. Effects of meloxicam and indomethacin on cyclooxygenase pathways in healthy volunteers. J Invest Med. 1997; 45: 44–9.

9. Cipollone C, Ganci A, Panara MR, et al. Effects of nabumetone on prostanoid biosynthesis in man. Clin Pharmacol Ther. 1995; 58: 335–41.

10. Emori WE, Champion GD, Bluestone R, Paulus HE. Simultaneous pharmacokinetics of indomethacin in serum and synovial fluid. Ann Rheum. Dis. 1983; 32: 433–5.

11. Fowler PD, Shadforth MF, Crook PR, John VA. Plasma and synovial fluid concentrations of diclofenac sodium and its major hydroxylated metabolites during long-term treatment of rheumatoid arthritis. Eur J Clin Pharmacol. 1983; 25: 389–94.

12. Fowler PD, Dawes PT, John VA, Shotton PA. Plasma and synovial fluid concentrations of diclofenac sodium and its hydroxylated metabolites during once daily administration of a 100 mg slow-release formulation. Eur J Clin Pharmacol. 1986; 31: 469–72.

13. Kurowski M, Dunky A. Transsynovial kinetics of piroxicam in patients with rheumatoid arthritis. Eur J Clin Pharmacol. 1988; 34: 401–6.

14. Türck D, Busch, U, Heinzel G, Narjes H. Clinical pharmacokinetics of meloxicam. Arzneim-Forsch/Drug Res. 1997; 47: 253–8.

15. Day RO, Francis H, Vial J, Geisslinger G, Williams KM. Naproxen concentrations in plasma and synovial fluid and effects on prostanoid concentrations. J Rheumatol. 1995; 22: 2295–303.

16. Chérié Lignière G, Tamborini U, Panarace G. La nimesulide nel liquido sinoviale di pazienti con artrite reumatoide. Farm Tera. 1990; 7: 173–6.

17. Miehlke RK, Schneider S, Sorgel F et al. Penetration of the active metabolite of nabumetone into synovial fluid. Drugs. 1990; 40 (suppl 5): 57–61.

18. Schwinghammer TL, Kroboth PD. Basic concepts in pharmaco-dynamic modeling. J Clin Pharmacol. 1988; 28: 388–94.

19. Distel M, Mueller C, Bluhmki E, Fries J. Safety of meloxicam: a global analysis of safety clinical trials. Br J Rheumatol. 1996; 35 (Suppl 1): 68–77.

12 New highly selective COX-2 inhibitors

A. W. FORD-HUTCHINSON

Cyclooxygenase (prostaglandin G/H-synthase, COX) exists in two isoforms which have been termed COX-1 (constitutive enzyme) and COX-2 (an inducible enzyme)[1,2]. COX-1 has been cloned from a number of sources including man, the mouse and sheep[3-7]. COX-2 was originally identified as a phorbol ester-inducible early gene product in murine 3T3 cells and as a v-src-inducible gene product in chicken fibroblasts[8,9]. These proteins were recognized as novel cyclooxygenases by their homology to COX-1. Human COX-2 cDNA was subsequently cloned and shown to have 64% overall amino acid sequence identity to human COX-1[10]. Similarities between the two isoforms include the fact that both proteins contain (a) a signal peptide sequence, (b) a putative membrane anchoring domain, (c) a conserved active site containing an aspirin acetylation site and (d) a C-terminal STEL sequence which may be responsible for retaining the protein in the endoplasmic reticulum. The most significant differences between COX-2 and COX-1 are in their regulation as COX-2 can be induced transiently over a >50 fold range by a variety of inflammatory mediators[2] as well as stimuli such as hypoxia[11], synaptic excitation[12-14], injury[15] and laminar sheer stress[16], and simply by incubation of tissues in vitro[17]. This induction can be inhibited by glucocorticoids. Consistent with this, the gene structures in the 5' region are very different between the two enzymes[2].

The mechanism of action of non-steroidal anti-inflammatory drugs involves inhibition of COX[18,19]. In addition, inhibition of the production of prostaglandins (PGs) explains the anti-inflammatory, analgesic and anti-pyretic activity of these compounds as well as their ability to inhibit hormone-induced uterine contractions and certain types of cancer growth. It is also abundantly clear that non-steroid anti-inflammatory drugs (NSAIDs) have mechanism-based side effects which include induction of gastrointestinal lesions, effects on renal function in compromised individuals, increases in bleeding time, induction of NSAID-induced asthma and prolongation of gestation and labour. Thus, it is clear that prostanoids have both physiological and pathological effects. The hypothesis behind the development of selective COX-2 inhibitors is that the therapeutic usefulness of NSAIDs will be largely due to inhibition of inducible COX-2, while the side effect profile will be mainly due to inhibition of COX-1[1,20]. All the NSAIDs currently on the market in North America show no significant degree of selectivity for COX-2.

DEVELOPMENT OF COX-2 INHIBITORS

A number of COX-2 inhibitors have been developed and early efforts were aimed at modifying two original leads (see Figure 1): the Dupont compound, DuP 697 (**1**)[21] and the Taisho compound, NS 398 (**2**)[22]. The latter compound is in the sulide class which includes L-745,337 (**3**), which has been used in animal studies to test the COX-2 hypothesis[23–25]. DuP 697 has led to the development of a number of classes of tricyclic compounds. These include (a) 4-membered rings such as 2,3-diarylcyclobutenone (**4**)[26], (b) 5-membered rings such as thiazoles, thiadiazoles (**5**) and oxazoles[27]. The furonone (**6**) has been shown to reduce the number of polyps in ApcΔ[716–/–] knockout

Figure 1. Examples of selective COX-2 inhibitors described in the literature

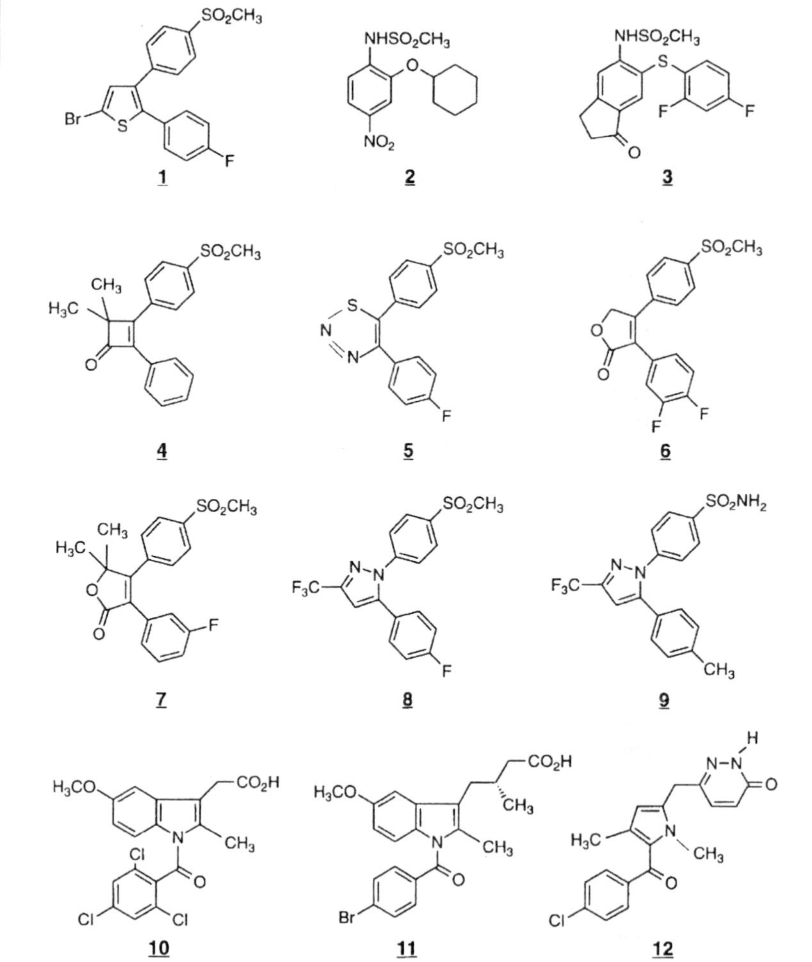

mice and together with data on crossbreeding with COX-2 knockout mice has been used to support the concept that COX-2 inhibition may retard intestinal polyp formation[28]. Compound (7) (DFU) has been reported to be a highly selective COX-2 inhibitor with activity in animal models of inflammation, pain and pyresis with no evidence for gastrointestinal erosions[29]. Other 5-membered rings include 1,5- diaryl pyrazole-based inhibitors such as SC-58125 (8) and celecoxib (9)[30]. (c) 6-membered rings using both benzene and pyridine rings[31] and (d) fused ring systems such as indoles and benzofurans[32].

Two groups have reported the development of selective COX-2 inhibitors from existing NSAIDs. Unlike all the above classes such compounds do not contain the SO_2R functionality. Utilizing differences in the sizes of the active site between COX-1 and COX-2, the 4-chlorobenzyl group of indomethacin was replaced with either a larger 2,4,6-trichlorobenzyl (10) or the 4-bromo group (11) and this led to COX-2 selective inhibitors[33,34]. Similarly replacement of the carboxylic acid group of Zomiperac with a pyridazinone moiety led to the development of selective inhibitors (12)[35].

MECHANISTIC STUDIES ON COX-2 INHIBITORS

Inhibition of COX-1 or COX-2 by potent inhibitors is time-dependent in both whole cell and cell-free assays. Upon mixing inhibitor and enzyme, the inhibition develops to its maximum level over a period ranging from minutes to hours. Increased inhibitor concentrations result in a faster development of inhibition. This behaviour is rationalized in terms of initial low affinity binding of the inhibitor in a rapidly reversible step, followed by a slower transition to a state in which the inhibitors are more tightly bound to the enzyme. This means that the fully developed time-dependent inhibition is only very slowly reversible. As inhibition of COX by most NSAIDs is believed to be competitive with substrate, increasing arachidonic acid concentrations will result in increases in the time required for the development of maximal inhibition of a time-dependent inhibitor.

The implications of this time-dependent inhibition are that inhibition of the enzyme target in vivo can persist even after plasma levels of the inhibitor have fallen well below that which is required for inhibition. In this case the duration of action of the drug may be limited more by the rate of de novo synthesis of the COX rather than by the pharmacokinetic parameters of the drug itself. This type of behaviour, however, is a significant liability for the development of selective COX-2 inhibitors. This is because rapid induction of COX-2 may result in the production of enzyme which is not exposed to inhibitor for a sufficient time before it begins acting upon a substrate. In such cases, the enzyme COX-2 might produce sufficient product before development of maximum inhibition, thus rendering the inhibition functionally ineffective.

Figure 2 shows the mechanism of action of selective COX-2 inhibitor on both COX-1 and COX-2[36,37]. Inhibition of COX-1 by selective COX-2 inhibitors is weak and time independent. Initially a selective COX-2 inhibitor will also function as a relatively weak, rapidly reversible inhibitor of COX-2. Maximum inhibition will

Figure 2. Kinetic mechanisms of cyclooxygenase inhibition by COX-2 inhibitors

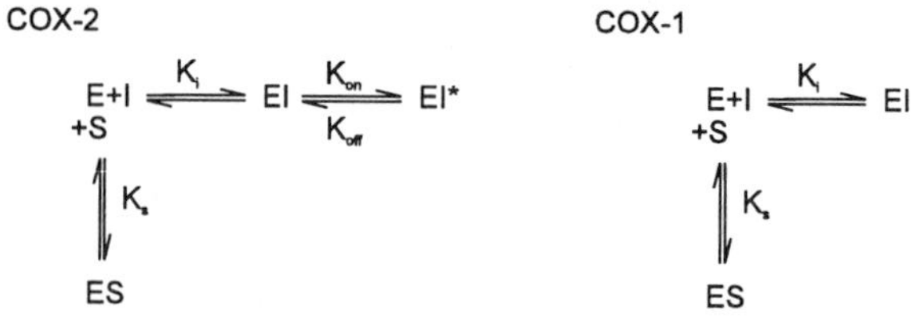

COX-2

$$E+I \; \underset{}{\overset{K_i}{\rightleftharpoons}} \; EI \; \underset{K_{off}}{\overset{K_{on}}{\rightleftharpoons}} \; EI^*$$
$$+S \; \Big\Updownarrow K_s$$
$$ES$$

COX-1

$$E+I \; \overset{K_i}{\rightleftharpoons} \; EI$$
$$+S \; \Big\Updownarrow K_s$$
$$ES$$

- Selectivity for COX-2 over COX-1 is achieved by the time-dependent formation of an essentially irreversible EI* complex

develop over a period of time, depending on the degree of time dependence of inhibition. Thus the selectivity of potent COX-2 inhibitors, which is only produced through this time-dependent interaction, will not be realized at early times after expression of COX-2. This will be particularly aggravated in acute inflammatory situations where high arachidonic concentrations may be present and which may result in an even smaller degree of functional selectivity. It is difficult to estimate the contribution of these factors to the in vivo selectivity and potency of selective COX-2 inhibitors. This mechanism serves to explain the wide variety of IC_{50} values obtained with different inhibitors under varying conditions of pre-incubation, enzyme concentrations and substrate concentrations and indicates that extremely high degrees of selectivity will be required to produce functional selectivity in vivo and hence reduction of COX-1 mediated side effects.

ANTI-INFLAMMATORY, ANALGESIC AND ANTI-PYRETIC ACTIVITIES OF COX-2 INHIBITORS

It is obviously of importance that selective COX-2 inhibitors should have equivalent anti-inflammatory, analgesic and anti-pyretic activity to mixed COX-1 and COX-2 inhibitors (NSAIDs). Studies carried out with the prototypic COX-2 inhibitor L-745,337 and other related COX-2 inhibitors have shown that in animal models these compounds produce similar reversals of pain and fever responses to indomethacin[23,24]. These compounds also showed anti-inflammatory activity comparable to NSAIDs in the rat carageenan paw oedema and the adjuvant arthritis models, which have proven to be predictive of activity in man[24,29]. These results do not exclude the possibility that in certain acute situations PGs may be released from constitutive COX-1, before induction of COX-2, and may contribute to early pain and inflammatory responses. On the other hand, it is also possible that the absence of mechanism-based side-effects with COX-2 inhibitors will allow for higher dosing in man leading to more complete suppression of PG production and hence to improved anti-inflammatory/analgesic activity. Preliminary data has been obtained in man with the highly COX-2 selective inhibitor, MK-966, a 4-methylsulphonylphenyl derivative. This compound produced equivalent inhibition of postoperative dental pain to that produced by Ibuprofen[38].

COX-2 INHIBITORS AND THEIR POTENTIAL FOR INDUCING GASTROINTESTINAL LESIONS

In the USA, NSAID usage has been estimated to result in 76000 hospitalizations and 7600 deaths per year[39]. This is consistent with the important physiological role for PGs within the gastrointestinal tract, where they appear to be involved in the control of gastric acid secretion, mucus production and maintenance of mucosal integrity and blood flow[40-43]. In the lower gastrointestinal tract PGs have been reported to have a role in the modulation of colonic motility, electrolyte and water secretion and proliferative activity within the colon[41,44]. Intestinal PGs may be produced from multiple cell types, including colonic and intestinal epithelial cells, immune cells in the lamina propria and subepithelial mesenchymal cells[45]. Following the discovery of COX-2, the expression of both COX-1 and COX-2 in the gastrointestinal tract of human and various animal species has been assessed. Widespread expression of COX-1 protein has been observed in a variety of gastrointestinal tissues from several species. In contrast, no expression of COX-2 proteins could be observed in most gastrointestinal tissues examined[46,47]. However, small amounts of COX-2 may be present in certain tissues, for example, in rat caecum[47], consistent with observations that COX-2 proteins in rat intestinal epithelial cells can be stimulated with transforming growth factor α. In contrast to the lack of expression of COX-2 in normal human intestinal tissues, significant levels of COX-2 expression have been observed in samples obtained from colon cancer tissues[46,48,49]. This has been interpreted as indicating that the protective effects of non-steroidal anti-inflammatory drug usage against colon cancer may be mediated by inhibition of COX-2.

Acute animal studies with selective prototypic COX-2 inhibitors demonstrates that such compounds lack the gastric toxicity associated with other NSAIDs. This has been demonstrated in studies with L-745,337 in rats and squirrel monkeys using chronic b.i.d. dosing over 4–5 days with subsequent monitoring of gastrointestinal damage through the faecal exretion of $^{51}CrCl_3$. Dramatic differences were observed between the selective COX-2 inhibitor and conventional NSAIDs with regard to the potential for inducing leakage in the gastrointestinal tract[24].

These observations in animals have also been extended to man in a study with the COX-2 selective inhibitor, MK-966. In this study healthy volunteers whose stomach and duodenum were free of either haemorrhage, erosion or ulcer as determined by endoscopy were treated for 7 days with either MK-966 250 mg once daily (a dose significantly greater than that required for the optimal relief of pain in patients with osteoarthritis), ibuprofen 800 mg t.i.d., aspirin 650 mg q.i.d. or placebo. Ibuprofen and aspirin produced significant numbers of stomach and/or duodenal lesions whereas MK-966 was similar to placebo[50].

COX-2 INHIBITORS AND PLATELET FUNCTION

Platelets have been shown to express only COX-1, and COX-2 protein cannot be detected by Western blot analysis. COX-2 inhibitors therefore have no effect on platelet thromboxane B_2 production and thus will have no effect on the aggregation of platelets induced by a variety of agents including collagen, ADP and thromboxane A_2. These results indicate that selective COX-2 inhibitors will not increase bleeding times as observed with conventional NSAIDs. NSAIDs are contraindicated in patients with gastrointestinal bleeding, coagulation disorders and other bleeding problems as well as in patients prior to surgery or those taking anticoagulants. It is possible that such restrictions may not be applicable to COX-2 selective compounds.

COX-2 INHIBITORS AND RENAL FUNCTION

Prostaglandins may have a significant modulatory role in the kidney through their effects on a variety of renal events including renin release, water and salt reabsorption, renal blood flow redistribution and the control of glomerular filtration and renal vascular resistance[51–53]. In patients with impaired kidney function, administration of NSAIDs induces a reduction in glomerular filtration rate which is associated with water and sodium retention and a decrease in renal blood flow. These patients can be classified into two groups. First, there are those with activation of systemic or renal vasoconstrictor systems (e.g. the sympathetic nervous system or angiotensin-II) including volume depletion, hypotension, congestive heart failure, nephrotic syndrome and hepatic cirrhosis with ascites, patent ductus arteriosus, etc. Secondly, there are those with diseases directly affecting the kidneys such as pyelonephritis and lupus nephritis. The first group are those where most of the 'unexpected' deterioration of renal function has occurred.

COX-1 is abundantly expressed throughout the kidney. Regulation of COX-2 has been observed in kidneys in the macula densa following salt deprivation[54]. Pharmacological studies in the rabbit have indicated that the increased or exaggerated PG production observed in hydronephrotic kidneys may be attributable to COX-2, whereas the basal release of PGs is attributable to COX-1[55]. These results suggest that the renal PG production in the normal kidney is driven by the activity of COX-1, while kidneys subject to either inflammatory or other challenges can show induction of COX-2. Detailed studies will be required in man to determine whether selective COX-2 inhibitors will possess some or all of the renal side effects associated with conventional NSAIDs.

CONCLUSIONS

Preclinical and early clinical data supports the hypothesis that selective COX-2 inhibitors will have anti-inflammatory, analgesic and anti-pyretic activities comparable to NSAIDs with a substantial reduction in some of the side effects associated with this class of drugs, particularly induction of gastric lesions and effects on bleeding times. The effects of selective COX-2 inhibitors on renal function in renally-compromised individuals remains to be determined. Mechanistic studies indicate that a high degree of in vitro biochemical selectivity for COX-2 will be required in order to achieve effective functional selectivity in vivo. A number of highly selective COX-2 inhibitors have been synthesized and described in the scientific and patent literature and early data are supportive of the concept that such compounds will represent an important therapeutic advance.

References

1. Smith WL, DeWitt DL. Biochemistry of prostaglandin endoperoxide H synthase-1 and synthase-2 and their differential susceptibility to nonsteroidal anti-inflammatory drugs. Semin Nephrol. 1995; 15: 179–94.
2. Herschman HR. Prostaglandin synthase 2. Biochim Biophys Acta. 1996; 1299: 125–40.
3. DeWitt DL, Smith WL. Primary structure of prostaglandin G/H synthase from sheep vesicular gland determined from the complementary DNA sequence. Proc Natl Acad Sci USA. 1988; 85: 1412–16.
4. Merlie JP, Fagan D, Mudd J, Needleman P. Isolation and characterization of the complementary DNA for sheep seminal vesicle prostaglandin endoperoxide synthase (cyclooxygenase). J Biol Chem. 1988; 263: 3550–3.
5. Yokoyama C, Takai T, Tanabe T. Primary structure of sheep prostaglandin endoperoxide synthase deduced from cDNA sequence. FEBS Lett. 1988; 231: 347–51.
6. DeWitt DL, el-Harith EA, Kraemer SA et al. The aspirin and heme-binding sites of ovine and murine prostaglandin endoperoxide synthases. J Biol Chem. 1990; 265: 5192–8.
7. Yokoyama C, Tanabe T. Cloning of human gene encoding prostaglandin endoperoxide synthase and primary structure of the enzyme. Biochem Biophys Res Commun. 1989; 165: 888–94.
8. Kujubu DA, Fletcher BS, Varnum BC, Lim RW, Herschman HR. TIS10, a phorbol ester tumor promoter-inducible mRNA from Swiss 3T3 cells, encodes a novel prostaglandin synthase/cyclooxygenase homologue. J Biol Chem. 1991; 266: 12866–72.
9. Xie WL, Chipman JG, Robertson DL, Erikson RL, Simmons DL. Expression of a mitogen-responsive gene encoding prostaglandin synthase is regulated by mRNA splicing. Proc Natl Acad Sci USA. 1991; 88: 2692–6.
10. Hla T, Neilson K. Human cyclooxygenase-2 cDNA. Proc Natl Acad Sci USA. 1992; 89: 7384–8.
11. Schmedtje JF Jr, Ji YS, Liu WL, Dubois RN, Runge, MS. Hypoxia induces cyclooxygenase-2 via the NF-kappa-B p65 transcription factor in human vascular endothelial cells. J Biol Chem. 1997; 272: 601–8.
12. Adams J, Collaco-Moraes Y, de Belleroche J. Cyclooxygenase-2 induction in cerebral cortex: An intracellular response to synaptic excitation. J Neurochem. 1996; 66: 6–13.
13. Kaufmann WE, Worley PF, Pegg J, Bremer M, Isakson P. COX-2, a synaptically induced enzyme, is expressed by excitatory neurons at postsynaptic sites in rat cerebral cortex. Proc Natl Acad Sci USA. 1996; 93: 2517–21.
14. Marcheselli VL, Bazan NG. Sustained induction of prostaglandin endoperoxide synthase-2 by seizures in hippocampus: Inhibition by a platelet-activating factor antagonist. J Biol Chem. 1996; 271: 24794–9.
15. Pritchard KA Jr, O'Banion MK, Miana JM et al. Induction of cyclooxygenase-2 in rat vascular smooth muscles in vitro and in vivo. J Biol Chem. 1994; 269: 8504–9.
16. Topper JN, Cai J, Falb D, Gimbrone MA. Identification of vascular endothelial genes differentially responsive to fluid mechanical stimuli: Cyclooxygenase-2, manganese superoxide dismutase and endothelial cell nitric oxide synthase are selectively up-regulated by steady laminar shear stress. Proc Natl Acad Sci USA. 1996; 93: 10417–22.
17. Charette L, Misquitta C, Guay J, Riendeau D, Jones TR. Involvement of cyclooxygenase-2 (COX-2) in intrinsic tone of isolated guinea pig trachea. Can J Physiol Pharmacol. 1995; 73: 1561–7.
18. Vane JR. Inhibition of prostaglandin synthesis as a mechanism of action for aspirin-like drugs. Nature New Biol. 1971; 231: 232–5.
19. Flower RJ, Vane JR. Inhibition of prostaglandin biosynthesis. Biochem Pharmacol. 1974; 23: 1439–50.
20. Vane JR, Botting RM. New insights into the mode of action of anti-inflammatory drugs. Inflammation Res. 1995; 44: 1–10.

21. Gans KR, Galbraith W, Roman RJ et al. Anti-inflammatory and safety profile of DuP697, a novel orally effective prostaglandin synthesis inhibitor. J Pharmacol Exp Ther. 1990; 254: 180–7.
22. Futaki N, Takahashi S, Yokoyama M, Arai I, Higuchi S, Otomo S. NS-398, a new anti-inflammatory agent, selectively inhibits prostaglandin G/H synthase/cyclooxygenase (COX-2) activity in vitro. Prostaglandins. 1994; 47: 55–9.
23. Boyce S, Chan CC, Gordon R et al. L-745,337: a selective inhibitor of cyclooxygenase-2 elicits antinociception but not gastric ulceration in rats. Neuropharmacology. 1994; 33: 1609–11.
24. Chan CC, Boyce S, Brideau C et al. Pharmacology of a selective cyclooxygenase-2 inhibitor, L-745,337: A novel nonsteroidal anti-inflammatory agent with an ulcerogenic sparing effect in rat and nonhuman primate stomach. J Pharmacol Exp Ther. 1995; 274: 1531–7.
25. Prasit P, Black WC, Chan CC et al. L-745,337, a selective cyclooxygenase-2 inhibitor. Med Chem Res. 1995; 5: 364–74.
26. Friesen RW, Dubé D, Fortin R et al. Novel 1,2-diarylcyclobutenes: Selective and orally active COX-2 inhibitors. Bioorg Med Chem Lett. 1996; 6: 2677–82.
27. Gauthier JY, Leblanc Y, Black WC et al. Synthesis and biological evaluation of 2,3-diarylthiophenes as selective COX-2 inhibitors Part II: Replacing the heterocycle. Bioorg Med Chem Lett. 1996; 6: 87–92.
28. Oshima M, Dinchuk JE, Kargman SL et al. Suppression of intestinal polyposis in Apc Delta-716 knockout mice by inhibition of cyclooxygenase 2 (COX-2). Cell. 1996; 87: 803–9.
29. Riendeau D, Percival MD, Boyce S et al. Biochemical and pharmacological profile of a tetrasubstituted furanone as a highly selective COX-2 inhibitor. Br J Pharmacol. 1997; 121: 105–17.
30. Penning TD, Talley JJ, Bertenshaw SR et al. Synthesis and biological evaluation of the 1,5-diarylpyrazole class of cyclooxygenase-2 inhibitors: Identification of 4-[5-(4-methyl phenyl-3-trifluoromethyl)-1H-pyrazol-1-yl] benzenesulfonamide(SC-58635, Celecoxib). J Med Chem. 1997; 40: 1347–65.
31. Li JJ, Norton MB., Reinhard EJ et al. Novel terphenyls as selective cyclooxygenase-2 inhibitors and orally active anti-inflammatory agents. J Med Chem. 1996; 39: 1846–56.
32. Huang HC, Chamberlain TS, Seibert K, Koboldt CM, Isakson PC, Reitz DB. Diaryl indenes and benzofurans: novel class of potent and selective cyclooxygenase-2 inhibitors. Bioorg Med Chem Lett., 1995; 5: 2377–80.
33. Black WC, Bayly C, Belley M et al. From indomethacin to a selective COX-2 inhibitor: development of indolakanoic acids as potent and selective cyclooxygenase-2 inhibitors. Bioorg Med Chem Lett. 1996; 6: 725–30.
34. Leblanc Y, Black WC, Chan CC et al. Synthesis and biological evaluation of both enantiomers of L-761,000 as inhibitors of cyclooxygenase 1 and 2. Bioorg Med Chem Lett. 1996; 6: 73.
35. Barnett JW, Dunn JP, Kertesz DJ et al. Pyrrole derivatives. European Patent, 714895. 1996, June 5.
36. Ouellet M, Percival DM. Effect of inhibitor time-dependency on selectivity towards cyclooxygenase isoforms. Biochem J. 1995; 306: 247–51.
37. Copeland RA, Williams JM, Giannaras J et al. Mechanism of selective inhibition of the inducible isoform of prostaglandin G/H synthase. Proc Natl Acad Sci USA. 1994; 91: 11202–6.
38. Ehrich E, Mehlisch D, Perkins S et al. Efficacy of MK-966, a highly selective inhibitor of COX-2, in the treatment of postoperative dental pain. Arthritis Rheum. 1996; 39 (Suppl 9): S81.
39. Fries JF. NSAID gastropathy: the second most deadly rheumatic disease? Epidemiology and risk approval. J Rheumatol. S 1991; 28 (Suppl.): 6–10.
40. Sandor Z, Szabo S. Pharmacological approaches and pathogenic basis of NSAID gastropathy: Prevention and treatment. Pract Gastroenterol. 1991; 15: 30–43.
41. Robert A, Ruwart M. Effects of prostaglandins on the digestive system. In: Lee JB (ed.). Prostaglandins. New York: Elsevier North Holland, 1982: 113–76.
42. Fletcher JR. Eicosanoids. Arch Surg. 1993; 128: 1192–6.

43. Wallace JL. Prostaglandins, NSAIDS, and cytoprotection. Gastroenterol Clin North Am. 1992; 21: 631–41.
44. Bennett A. Prostaglandins and the alimentary tract. In: Karim SMM (ed.). Prostaglandins: Physiological, Pharmacological and Pathological Aspects. Baltimore: University Press, 1976: 247–76.
45. Eberhart CE, DuBois RN. Eicosanoids and the gastrointestinal tract. Gastroenterology. 1995; 109: 285–301.
46. Kargman SL, O'Neill GP, Vickers PJ, Evans JF, Mancini JA, Jothy S. Expression of prostaglandin G/H synthase-1 and -2 protein in human colon cancer. Cancer Res. 1995; 55: 2556–9.
47. Kargman S, Charleson S, Cartwright M, et al. Prostaglandin G/H synthase-1 and -2 in rat, dog, monkey and human gastrointestinal tracts: Localization, enzymatic activity and inhibition by NSAIDS. Gastroenterology. In press.
48. Eberhart CE, Coffey RJ, Radhika A, Giardiello FM, Ferrenbach S, Dubois RN. Upregulation of cyclooxygenase 2 gene expression in human colorectal adenomas and adenocarcinomas. Gastroenterology 1994; 107: 1183–8.
49. Sano H, Kawahito Y, Wilder RL et al. Expression of cyclooxygenase-1 and -2 in human colorectal cancer. Cancer Res. 1995; 55: 3785–9.
50. Lanza F, Simon T, Quan H et al. Selective inhibition of cyclooxygenase-2 (COX-2) with MK-0966 (250mg Q.D.) is associated with less gastrointestinal damage than aspirin (ASA) 650mg Q.I.D. or ibuprofen (IBU) 800mg T.I.D. Gastroenterology. 1997, 112: A194.
51. Clive DM, Stoff JS. Renal syndromes associated with nonsteroidal anti-inflammatory drugs. N Engl J Med. 1984; 310: 563–72.
52. Jackson EK, Branch RA, Margolius HS, Oates JA. Physiological functions of the renal prostaglandin, renin and kallikrein systems. In: Seldin DW, Giebisch G (eds). The Kidney: Physiology and Pathophysiology. New York: Raven; 1985: 613–36.
53. Murray MD, Brater DC. Renal toxicity of the nonsteroidal anti-inflammatory drugs. Annu Rev Pharmacol Toxicol. 1993; 33: 435–65.
54. Harris RC, McKanna JA, Akai Y, Jacobson HR, Dubois RN. Cyclooxygenase-2 is associated with the macula densa of rat kidney and increased with salt restriction. J Clin Invest 1994; 94: 2504–10.
55. Seibert K, Masferrer JL, Needleman P, Salvemini D. Pharmacological manipulation of cyclo-oxygenase-2 in the inflamed hydronephrotic kidney. Br J Pharmacol. 1996; 117: 1016–20.

13 Specific COX-2 inhibitors: from bench to bedside

P. ISAKSON, B. ZWEIFEL, J. MASFERRER,
C. KOBOLDT, K. SEIBERT, R. HUBBARD,
S. GEIS and P. NEEDLEMAN

Non-steroidal anti-inflammatory drugs (NSAIDs) such as aspirin have been used to treat various ailments for over 100 years. As a class, these drugs are anti-inflammatory, analgesic and anti-pyretic, and they are widely used to treat chronic inflammatory diseases such as arthritis. The commercially available NSAIDs are approximately equivalent in terms of anti-inflammatory efficacy. All of the NSAIDs, however, also cause adverse effects in a significant fraction of people who consume them, and these side-effects frequently limit therapy. The most common side-effects associated with NSAID therapy are gastrointestinal (GI), with haemorrhage and frank ulceration seen in some patients; these lesions apparently can lead to increased morbidity in long-term NSAID users[1]. Renal and CNS effects are also observed. Because of these problems, a major goal of the pharmaceutical industry is the development of drugs that possess anti-inflammatory activity but lack the toxic effects associated with current NSAIDs. To date, no NSAIDs with the desired therapeutic profile have been commercially developed.

A biochemical mechanism of action for NSAIDs was discovered in the early 1970s, when these drugs were found to inhibit the enzyme cyclooxygenase (COX), thus preventing the production of prostaglandins (PGs)[2,3]. Most cells and tissues produce PGs, and they have a diverse array of biological functions. Of particular note are the cytoprotective actions of PGs in the gastrointestinal (GI) tract, and the effects of PGs on renal and platelet function. In addition to these important roles in normal physiology, PGs are also associated with inflammatory conditions[4] and have been shown to cause many of the signs and symptoms of inflammation including oedema, hyperaemia and hyperalgesia[4,5]. For many years it was believed that PGs were formed via the activity of a single enzyme COX, that is present constitutively in most cells[4]. Inhibition of COX would lead to decreased production of pro-inflammatory PGs at the site of inflammation while at the same time inhibit the formation of PGs that play a role in sustaining normal cellular or tissue function. A corollary of this view was that the availability of substrate arachidonic acid was the sole means of regulating PG production. This view was challenged by a number of experiments demonstrating that the amount of COX enzyme was regulated in inflammatory conditions. One of the first such observations was in a rabbit model of hydronephrosis, characterized by markedly elevated PG production following ureter obstruction[6]. Exaggerated PG production in this model was associated with an influx in inflammatory cells such as macrophages and fibroblasts, and with an increase in the mass of COX enzyme[6,7]. In vitro experiments then demonstrated that incubation of fibroblasts or monocytes with the inflammatory cytokine IL-1 caused a similar increase in PG synthetic capacity that was associated with elevated amounts of COX enzyme; importantly, increases in PG synthetic capacity and COX enzyme levels were inhibited by the anti-inflammatory glucocorticoid dexamethasone, but this drug did not alter basal COX activity observed in vitro or in vivo[8–11]. Based on these data it was hypothesized that there is an inducible form of the COX enzyme that was sensitive to cytokine stimulation and selective inhibition by glucocorticoids. Furthermore, lowering endogenous glucocorticoids by adrenalectomy increased levels of COX in macrophages[9]. The hypothesis that a regulated form of COX existed was supported by the isolation of a second COX gene whose expression is induced by a number of inflammatory cytokines, and selectively blocked by dexamethasone[12–21].

The two COX genes are clearly closely related and contain stretches of near identity. All of the commercially available NSAIDs inhibit both forms of the enzyme at approximately the same concentrations (discussed more fully below). Comparison of the active sites of the two enzymes by X-ray crystallography[22,23] demonstrates that the active sites of the two enzymes are very similar, differing by a single residue out of 25. Mutation of that residue in COX-2 was shown to alter the inhibitor profile to one similar to COX-1[24]. The close similarity of the two enzymes might suggest that it would be difficult to selectively inhibit one of the enzymes. However, several compounds have now been described in the literature that show a high degree of selectivity for COX-2, including DuP 697, NS 398, flosulide, SC-58125 and L-745,337[25–27]. These compounds are equivalent to non-selective NSAIDs in anti-inflammatory, analgesic and anti-pyretic activity, but do not cause formation of gastrointestinal lesions typical of the NSAIDs[28–30]. These data suggest a model for the distribution and function of COX-1 and COX-2 as depicted in Figure 1.

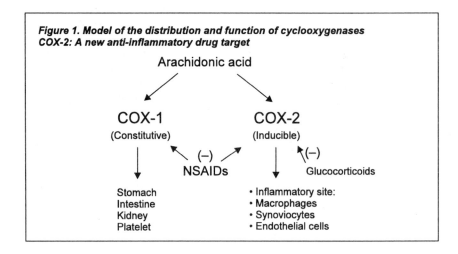

Figure 1. Model of the distribution and function of cyclooxygenases
COX-2: A new anti-inflammatory drug target

SC-58635, A SELECTIVE COX-2 INHIBITOR

Based on the pharmacological profile mentioned above, we hypothesized that a selective COX-2 inhibitor would be an efficacious anti-inflammatory and analgesic agent with an inherently superior safety profile compared to NSAIDs, particularly with regard to gastrointestinal safety. We therefore embarked on a program to identify selective COX-2 inhibitors suitable for evaluation of this hypothesis in man. This effort led to the discovery of SC-58635 or celecoxib, a compound with high selectivity for COX-2 (Table 1)[31].

Table 1. Celecoxib is highly selective for COX-2 and is ulcerogenic only in doses many times higher than those effective in inflammatory disease models

	IC_{50} (μM)		ED_{50} (mg/kg)		
	COX-1	COX-2	Carrageenan oedema	Adjuvant arthritis	GI ulcers
Indomethacin	0.2	1.2	2	0.1	8
SC-58635 (celecoxib)	15	0.04	10	0.3	>600

As can be seen in Table 1, celecoxib is a potent and selective inhibitor of COX-2, with activity in standard rodent models of inflammation and pain[31], but which lacks acute GI toxicity. Although the high degree of selectivity observed in the enzyme assay is important, it is but one aspect of the data needed to establish a unique safety profile. There has been considerable debate among those involved in this field concerning the interpretation of selectivity ratios (i.e. half-maximal inhibitory concentrations on COX-1/COX-2) and the appropriate (i.e. predictive) in vitro assay for determining these ratios. The difficulties in interpreting in vitro data are compounded by the complex mechanism by which most compounds inhibit either COX-1 or COX-2. Thus, most of the NSAIDs, including such drugs as diclofenac and indomethacin, inhibit both isoforms in a time-dependent, pseudo-irreversible fashion first described by Lands[32]. Although a competitive component to this inhibition is present (typically high micromolar affinity), the potency of these drugs as inhibitors derives from the time-dependent binding (low nanomolar inhibition). Selectivity for COX-2 occurs by retention of the high affinity time-dependent binding to COX-2 but only the competitive component of binding on COX-1[33,34] With such a complex mechanism of enzyme inhibition, one might predict that the results of in vitro enzyme essays would be highly dependent on such variables as enzyme and substrate concentration, presence or absence of membranes, and time and order of addition of substrate and inhibitor; such is indeed the case leading to remarkably divergent values for intrinsic potency, and COX-1/COX-2 inhibitor ratios[35]. For example we have found that varying the incubation time of enzyme with arachidonic acid (enzyme pre-incubated with inhibitor) can markedly affect the selectivity of marketed NSAIDs (data not shown). As shown in Figure 2, the relative selectivity of celecoxib on COX-1 and COX-2 is not appreciably affected by incubation time with arachidonic acid, suggesting relatively tight binding of inhibitor to enzyme.

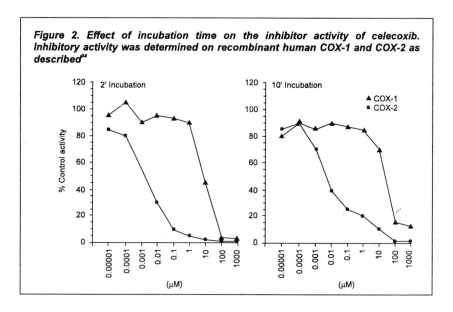

Figure 2. Effect of incubation time on the inhibitor activity of celecoxib. Inhibitory activity was determined on recombinant human COX-1 and COX-2 as described[24]

With the inherent complexities noted above, our approach has been to use the in vitro enzyme assay to guide further medicinal chemistry, but to develop in vivo assays capable of assessing biochemical efficacy in relevant tissues. For COX-1 activity, we have focused on the gastric mucosa, as the GI tract is clearly important from a therapeutic safety aspect, and it has been established that PGs in the GI tract are derived almost exclusively from COX-1[28,36]. The carrageenan induced air pouch in the rat has been developed as an assay for in vivo COX-2 activity. The air pouch model is a convenient source of inflammatory PGs, as the exudate can be readily sampled and has high PG levels, and it has been demonstrated to be driven by COX-2[28]. Thus, PG production associated with either COX-1 or COX-2 can be assessed after dosing animals, and half maximal inhibitory doses (ID_{50}) can be determined. Representative data with celecoxib is shown in Figure 3.

Efficacy of celecoxib in man

The data presented thus far suggest that celecoxib possesses a unique efficacy and safety profile in pre-clinical studies compared to all of the marketed NSAIDs; it is our hypothesis that this remarkable profile is due to the intrinsic ability of this compound to specifically inhibit COX-2 at therapeutic blood levels. While the pre-clinical data may be compelling, for this hypothesis to be truly borne out, equivalent data must be generated in man. Our Phase II studies were aimed at determining whether celecoxib was efficacious in arthritis and pain, and whether it affected COX-1 at therapeutic or higher blood levels. The results of those studies (Simon et al., submitted) demonstrated that celecoxib: (1) was efficacious in rheumatoid arthritis at doses of 200 and 400 mg b.i.d.; (2) was efficacious in osteoarthritis at doses ranging from 40 to 200 mg b.i.d.; (3) was efficacious in post-surgical dental pain at doses ranging from 50 to 400 mg;

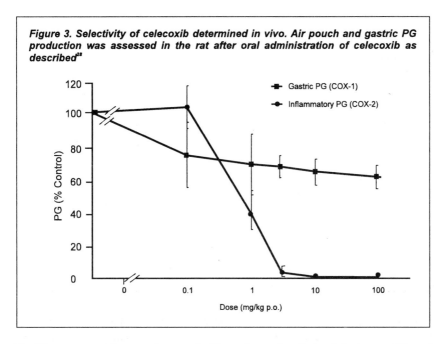

Figure 3. Selectivity of celecoxib determined in vivo. Air pouch and gastric PG production was assessed in the rat after oral administration of celecoxib as described[28]

(4) did not cause ulcers or increased GI erosions after 7 days' dosing at 100 and 200 mg b.i.d. Naproxen at 500 mg b.i.d. caused ulcers in nearly 20% of subjects; (5) did not affect platelet aggregation or thromboxane B_2 production in subjects dosed up to 600 mg b.i.d. for 6 days.

While the exact dose to be used therapeutically cannot be judged with precision from these data, the results of Phase II studies suggest that celecoxib is efficacious in arthritis and pain, and that at therapeutic doses it did not cause GI lesions that are typical of NSAIDs. The data with platelets is particularly striking in that doses well out of the predicted therapeutic range, which achieved proportionally high plasma levels, had no effect on platelet COX-1.

In conclusion, the pre-clinical and clinical data with celecoxib suggest that selective COX-2 inhibitors will have the efficacy profile of current NSAIDs without their GI and platelet side effects, thus providing good evidence to support the hypothesis outlined above. If phase III studies confirm this conclusion a new era of therapy for the arthritic diseases will have begun.

References

1. Allison MC, Howatson AG, Torrance CJ, Lee FD, Russell R. Gastrointestinal damage associated with the use of nonsteroidal antiinflammatory drugs. New England J Med. 1992; 327: 749–54.
2. Vane JR. Inhibition of prostaglandin synthesis as a mechanism of action for the aspirin-like drugs. Nature New Biol. 1971; 231: 232–5.
3. Smith JB, Willis AL. Aspirin selectively inhibits prostaglandin formation in human platelets. Nature New Biol. 1971; 231: 235–9.

4. Vane JR, Botting RM. Biological properties of cyclooxygenase products. In: Cunningham FM (ed.) Lipid Mediators. London: Academic Press Ltd, 1994; 61–97.
5. Portanova J, Zhang Y, Anderson GD et al. Selective neutralization of prostaglandin E_2 blocks inflammation, hyperalgesia and IL-6 production in vivo. J Exp Med. 1996; 184: 883–91.
6. Morrison AR, Nishikawa KA, Needleman P. Unmasking of thromboxane A2 synthesis by ureteral obstruction in the rabbit kidney. Nature. 1977; 267: 259–60.
7. Needleman P, Wyche A, Bronson SD, Holmberg S, Morrison AR. J Biol Chem. 1979; 254: 9772–7.
8. Raz A, Wyche A, Siegel N, Needleman P. Temporal and pharmacological division of fibroblast cyclooxygenase expression into transcriptional and translational phases. Proc Natl Acad Sci USA. 1989; 86: 1657–61.
9. Masferrer JL, Seibert K, Zweifel BS, Needleman P. Endogenous glucocorticoids regulate an inducible cyclooxygenase enzyme. Proc Natl Acad Sci USA. 1992; 89: 3917–21.
10. Masferrer JL, Zweifel BS, Seibert K, Needleman P. Selective regulation of cellular cyclooxygenase by dexamethasone and endotoxin in mice. J Clin Invest. 1990; 86: 1375–9.
11. Merlie JP, Fagan D, Mudd J, Needleman P. Isolation and characterization of complementary DNA for sheep seminal vesicle sheep prostaglandin endoperoxide synthase. J Biol Chem. 1988; 263: 3550–3.
12. DeWitt D, Smith WL. Primary structure of prostaglandin G/H synthase from sheep vesicular gland determined from the complementary DNA sequence. Proc Natl Acad Sci USA. 1988; 85: 1412–16.
13. Yokoyama C, Takai T, Tanabe T. Primary structure of sheep prostaglandin endoperoxide synthase deduced from cDNA sequence. FEBS Lett. 1988; 231: 347–51.
14. Xie W, Chipman JG, Robertson DL, Erikson RL, Simmons DL. Expression of a mitogen-responsive gene encoding prostaglandin synthase is regulated by mRNA splicing. Proc Natl Acad Sci USA. 1991; 88: 2692–6.
15. Kujubu DA, Fletcher BS, Varnum BC, Lim RW, Herschman HR. TIS10, a phorbol ester tumor promoter-inducible mRNA from Swiss 3T3 cells, encodes a novel prostaglandin synthase/cyclooxygenase homologue. J Biol Chem. 1991; 266: 12866–72.
16. O'Banion MK, Sadowski HB, Winn V, Young DA. A serum- and glucocorticoid regulated 4-kilobase mRNA encodes a cyclooxygenase-related protein. J Biol Chem. 1991; 266: 23261–7.
17. Fletcher BS, Kujubu DA, Perrin DM, Herschman HR. Structure of the mitogen-inducible TIS10 gene and demonstration that the TIS10-encoded protein is a functional prostaglandin G/H synthase. J Biol Chem. 1992; 267: 4338–44.
18. Sirois J, Richards JS. Purification and characterization of a novel, distinct isoform of prostaglandin endoperoxide synthase induced by human chorionic gonadotropin in granulosa cells of rat preovulatory follicles. J Biol Chem. 1992; 267: 6382–8.
19. Kujubu DA, Herschman HR. Dexamethasone inhibits mitogen induction of the TIS10 prostaglandin synthase/cyclooxygenase gene. J Biol Chem. 1992; 267: 7991–4.
20. O'Banion MK, Winn V, Young DA. cDNA cloning and functional activity of a glucocorticoid-regulated inflammatory cyclooxygenase. Proc Natl Acad Sci USA. 1992; 89: 4888–92.
21. Kujubu DA, Reddy ST, Fletcher BS, Herschman H. Expression of the protein product of the prostaglandin synthase-2/TIS10 gene in mitogen-stimulated Swiss 3T3 cells. J Biol Chem. 1993; 268: 5425–30.
22. Picot D, Loll PJ, Garavito RM. The X-ray crystal structure of the membrane protein prostaglandin H_2 synthase-1. Nature. 1994; 367: 243–9.
23. Kurumbail RG, Stevens AM, Gierse JK et al. Structural basis for selective inhibition of cyclooxygenase-2 by anti-inflammatory agents. Nature. 1996; 384: 644–8.
24. Gierse J, McDonald J, Hauser S, Rangwala S, Seibert K. A single amino acid difference between cyclooxygenase-1 (COX-1) and -2 (COX-2) reverses the selectivity of COX-2 specific inhibitors. J Biol Chem. 1996; 271: 15810–14.
25. Futaki N, Arai I, Hamasaki S, Takahashi S, Higuchi S, Otomo S. Selective inhibition of NS-398 on prostanoid production in inflamed tissue in rat carrageenan-air-pouch inflammation. J Pharm Pharmacol. 1992; 45: 753–5.

26. Futaki N, Yoshikawa K, Yumiko H et al. NS-398, a novel non-steroidal anti-inflammatory drug with potent analgesic and antipyretic effect, which causes minimal stomach lesions. Gen Pharmacol. 1993; 24: 105–10.

27. Gans KR, Galbraith W, Roman RJ et al. Anti-inflammatory and safety profile of DuP 697; a novel orally effective prostaglandin synthesis inhibitor. J Pharmacol Exp Ther. 1989; 254: 180–7.

28. Masferrer J, Zweifel B, Manning PT et al. Selective inhibition of inducible cyclooxygenase 2 in vivo is anti-inflammatory and non-ulcerogenic. Proc Natl Acad Sci USA. 1994; 91: 3228–32.

29. Seibert K, Zhang Y, Leahy K et al. Pharmacological and biochemical demonstration of the role of cyclooxygenase 2 in inflammation and pain. Proc Natl Acad Sci USA. 1994; 91: 12013–7.

30. Chan C, Boyce S, Brideau C et al. Pharmacology of a selective cyclooxygenase-2 inhibitor, L-745,337: A novel nonsteroidal anti-inflammatory agent with an ulcerogenic sparing effect in rat and nonhuman primate stomach. J Pharm Exp Ther. 1995; 274: 1531–7.

31. Penning TD, Talley JJ, Bertenshaw SR et al. Synthesis and biological evaluation of the 1,5-diarylpyrazole class of cyclooxygenase-2 inhibitors: Identification of SC-58635 (celecoxib). J Med Chem. 1997; 40: 1347–65.

32. Rome LH, Lands WEM. Structural requirements for time-dependent inhibition of prostaglandin biosynthesis by anti-inflammatory drugs. Proc Natl Acad Sci USA. 1975; 72: 4863–5.

33. Copeland RA, Williams JM, Giannaras J et al. Mechanisms of selective inhibition of the inducible isoform of prostaglandin G/H synthase. Proc Natl Acad Sci USA. 1994; 91: 11202–6.

34. Gierse JK, Hauser SD, Creely DP et al. Expression and selective inhibition of the constitutive and inducible forms of human cyclooxygenase. Biochem J. 1995; 305: 479–84.

35. Frölich JC. A classification of NSAIDs according to the relative inhibition of cyclooxygenase isoenzymes. Trends Pharm Sci. 1997; 18: 30–4.

36. Kargman S, Charleson S, Cartwright M et al. Characterization of prostaglandin G/H synthase 1 and 2 in rat, dog, monkey, and human gastrointestinal tracts. Gastroenterology. 1996; 111: 445–54.

14 Meloxicam: selective COX-2 inhibition in clinical practice

D. E. FURST

The non-steroid anti-inflammatory drugs (NSAIDs) exert many of their effects through inhibition of the cyclooxygenase (COX) enzyme, thus preventing the formation of prostaglandins (PGs). COX exists in two isoforms: the constitutive COX-1 which is present in many tissues, particularly the stomach, kidneys, and platelets, and stimulates the physiological production of PGs; and the inducible COX-2, which is expressed in response to an inflammatory stimulus. Agents that selectively inhibit COX-2 have a theoretical advantage in that they should be potent inhibitors of the inflammatory response, but at the same time have a low potential for renal and gastric adverse effects. Meloxicam consistently shows selectivity towards COX-2.

COX-2 SELECTIVITY OF NSAIDs

The selectivity of an NSAID for the two COX isoforms may be described by the COX-2/COX-1 ratio, and a number of studies have been undertaken to compare the selectivity of meloxicam with other agents in clinical use. COX-2/COX-1 ratios are calculated from the IC_{50} values for both isoforms (the concentration of drug that inhibits prostaglandin synthesis by 50%),[1] but these values vary greatly depending on the assay systems used (Table 1). In order to assess fully the relative selectivity of different agents, assays have been performed using a number of different systems. Absolute values obtained in different systems vary considerably, but the rank order of COX-2/COX-1 ratios is generally similar over a wide variety of models.

Meloxicam has been compared with other agents in in vitro and ex vivo human cell assays and in in vivo assays of renal function and platelet aggregation. Meloxicam has consistently shown selectivity for COX-2, although it retains some activity against COX-1. This may have clinical implications, as there is some evidence that COX-1 plays a part in mediating the inflammatory response[1], and an agent with some activity against both COX-2 and COX-1 may be a better anti-inflammatory compound than a 'pure' COX-2 inhibitor.

In an in vitro microsomal assay system[4], meloxicam exhibited greater COX-2 selectivity than nimesulide (the only other agent under test that could be described as having some selectivity towards COX-2), whereas diclofenac was approximately equipotent against both COX isoforms and ibuprofen, naproxen, indomethacin, and 6-MNA (6-methoxynaphthylacetic acid, the active metabolite of nabumetone) all preferentially inhibited COX-1. Another assay performed by the same investigators used cells transfected with human COX isoforms[8], and again meloxicam was a more potent inhibitor of COX-2 than nimesulide. Piroxicam and diclofenac were equipotent

135

Table 1. COX-2/COX-1 inhibition by NSAIDs (IC_{50} ratio)*. Assay dependent differences (*higher values denote less COX-2 selectivity)[2-7]

	Diclofenac	Etodolac	Ibuprofen	Indomethacin	Meloxicam	6-MNA	Piroxicam
Guinea-pig macrophages stimulated vs unstimulated	2.2	–	–	30	0.33	–	33
Mouse recombinant enzyme transfected cos-cells	–	–	0.67	22	–	0.14	9.5
Human recombinant enzyme microsomal assay	0.5	–	5.7	3.5	0.013	na (m>3)	–
	1.5	0.09	–	5.7	–	na (n≥1)	–
Human recombinant enzyme transfected cos-cells	0.33	–	7.0	1.6	0.067	36	0.49
Human whole blood assays	0.33	0.12	4.6	3.0	–	–	0.23
	–	–	2	0.53	0.09	0.67	0.33

na = not applicable due to very low activity; 6-MNA = 6-methoxynaphthylacetic acid against both COX isoforms, while ibuprofen, naproxen, 6-MNA, indomethacin, and aspirin all preferentially inhibited COX-1. Finally, an assay using whole blood taken from healthy volunteers once again indicated that meloxicam was selective towards COX-2, while retaining some activity against COX-1[8,9]. By contrast, indomethacin and 6-MNA inhibited both isoforms to a similar degree, and S- and R-indobufen were selective towards COX-1.

Initial studies with meloxicam in healthy volunteers provided evidence that in vitro COX-2 selectivity translates into significant differences on COX-mediated functions in vivo. When compared with indomethacin (25 mg three times daily), meloxicam (7.5 mg once daily) was found to have no effect on either of two COX-1 mediated actions, renal excretion of prostaglandin E_2 (PGE_2) and platelet aggregation, whereas indomethacin inhibited both to a significant degree[10].

EFFICACY IN OSTEOARTHRITIS

The short-term equivalence of meloxicam and diclofenac in osteoarthritis (OA) was established in the Melissa trial, a four-week, double-blind, randomized trial comparing meloxicam 7.5 mg daily with slow release (SR) diclofenac 100 mg daily in a total of over 9000 patients in 26 countries (unpublished data). The study showed equivalence in mean reduction of pain on movement between the two groups over the course of the trial. In a longer, 6-month study of the same doses of these two agents in OA, meloxicam remained as effective as diclofenac[11].

In order to compare the efficacy of meloxicam with other newer NSAIDs, the literature was examined for comparable trials with etodolac and nabumetone. Four trials were identified which measured etodolac efficacy[12,13] and three trials which measured nabumetone efficacy[14]. The entrance criteria for all the NSAID trials were approximately equivalent, with well defined OA, standard double-blind design and comparable outcome measures with respect to patient assessment of pain and global OA activity. The graphic combination of these trials allows one to compare these NSAIDs in a qualitative (although not quantitative) manner[11-14]. In four separate double-blind trials, over 6–12 weeks, etodolac 600 mg/day was compared with diclofenac 150 mg/day, piroxicam 20 mg/day, naproxen 1000 mg/day[12], or nimesulide 200 mg/day[13]. In all four trials, etodolac produced statistically significant improvements in primary efficacy variables, with efficacy equivalent to that of the comparators. In three double-blind studies of up to 6 months' duration, a total of 496 patients with OA received nabumetone 1000 mg daily; comparators were naproxen 500 mg/day, aspirin 3600 mg/day, or placebo[14]. Nabumetone was significantly ($p \leq 0.01$) more effective than placebo and had comparable efficacy to naproxen or aspirin in the physicians' and patients' assessment of degree of pain and overall OA activity. These seven trials[12-14] were combined with a meloxicam trial involving 336 patients[11]. The meloxicam trial was also double-blind, of six months' duration and compared diclofenac 100 mg daily to meloxicam 7.5 mg daily. This 'cross-NSAID' comparison showed meloxicam to have efficacy approximately equal to that of diclofenac and etodolac 600 mg (Figure 1)[11,12,14].

Caution is required in interpreting these results because the disease activity in the

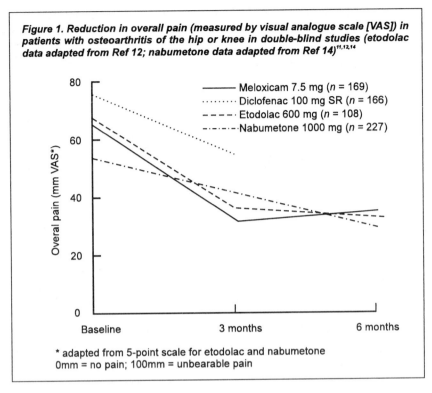

Figure 1. Reduction in overall pain (measured by visual analogue scale [VAS]) in patients with osteoarthritis of the hip or knee in double-blind studies (etodolac data adapted from Ref 12; nabumetone data adapted from Ref 14)[11,12,14]

Meloxicam 7.5 mg (n = 169)
Diclofenac 100 mg SR (n = 166)
Etodolac 600 mg (n = 108)
Nabumetone 1000 mg (n = 227)

* adapted from 5-point scale for etodolac and nabumetone
0mm = no pain; 100mm = unbearable pain

nabumetone trial was lower than it was in the patients in the meloxicam trial, while it was higher in the etodolac trial. By 'normalizing' the baselines and examining the slopes of change among the studies, etodolac 600 mg appears approximately equivalent to meloxicam 7.5 mg, while nabumetone 1000 mg daily appears to be numerically less effective than either meloxicam 7.5 mg or diclofenac 100 mg (no statistical testing was done). Indeed, in one study nabumetone 1000 mg daily was no more effective than placebo in OA of the knee, although it was effective in other settings[14]. Nabumetone is commonly used in US clinical practice at doses of 1500–2000 mg daily, a higher dose than was used in this study.

EFFICACY IN RHEUMATOID ARTHRITIS

Studies in rheumatoid arthritis (RA) have demonstrated that meloxicam is as effective as other NSAIDs. Meloxicam 7.5 mg (n = 199) was as effective as naproxen 750 mg (n = 180) daily for the treatment of RA over a period of 6 months[15]. In this trial there was a statistically significant difference in safety and tolerability favouring meloxicam. Twice as many patients taking naproxen withdrew from the trial because of gastrointestinal (GI) side effects as those taking meloxicam (12.2% vs 6%, respectively).

A higher dose of meloxicam, 15 mg daily, was compared with piroxicam 20 mg daily in RA[16]. A similar result was obtained, with no significant difference in the efficacy of the two agents but numerically (not statistically) more GI adverse events in the piroxicam group (14% vs 11%, respectively).

SAFETY OF MELOXICAM

Gastrointestinal safety and tolerability

The effect of meloxicam and piroxicam on the gastric mucosa has been directly studied by oesophagogastroduodenoscopy and monitoring of faecal blood loss[17]. In this double-blind, placebo-controlled trial, meloxicam in dosages of 7.5 mg and 15 mg daily was compared with both placebo and piroxicam 20 mg daily. Using the Lanza scoring system, the degree of GI damage was compared over the four-week trial (a somewhat shorter trial than now recommended). At the end of the study, the mean total endoscopic score in subjects taking piroxicam was significantly higher than in those taking either placebo or meloxicam 7.5 mg. Meloxicam 7.5 mg caused no significant change in the mucosal appearance. Six (50%) of the subjects taking piroxicam were withdrawn from the trial early because of deterioration in the endoscopic appearance of the gastric mucosa, whereas none of the meloxicam subjects (either dose) were withdrawn. With piroxicam, there was a significantly higher number of endoscopically detected ulcers developing during the study compared with the meloxicam 15 mg group (Figure 2).

The Melissa trial (unpublished data) also provided information about the GI safety of meloxicam 7.5 mg daily, compared with diclofenac 100 mg daily. During this large 4-week trial, GI side effects were significantly more common in the diclofenac group

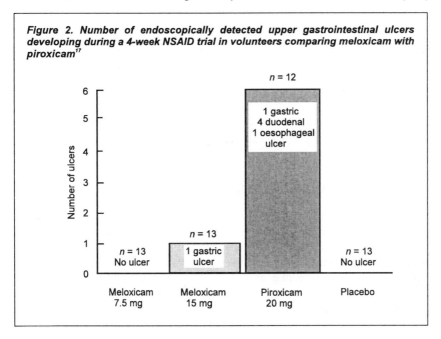

Figure 2. Number of endoscopically detected upper gastrointestinal ulcers developing during a 4-week NSAID trial in volunteers comparing meloxicam with piroxicam[17]

(19%) than in the meloxicam group (13%, $p < 0.001$). When individual symptoms were considered separately, diclofenac caused significantly more dyspepsia, abdominal pain, nausea and vomiting, and diarrhoea than meloxicam. The number of peptic ulcers and GI bleeds did not vary significantly between the groups, but this was as expected in a trial of 4 weeks' duration.

Extensive information about the GI safety of meloxicam and other NSAIDs in clinical use has been collected from a global analysis of the clinical trials programme, including a total of over 5600 patients in double-blind trials[18]. This represents 172 patient-years of exposure to meloxicam 7.5 mg, 1146 for meloxicam 15 mg, 166 for piroxicam 20 mg, 81 for diclofenac 100 mg, and 78 for naproxen 750–1000 mg. As a percentage (not accounting for duration of use) gastrointestinal side effects were most common in patients taking naproxen 750–1000 mg daily, followed (in order of decreasing frequency) by diclofenac 100 mg daily, piroxicam 20 mg daily, meloxicam 15 mg daily, and meloxicam 7.5 mg daily (Table 2).

Table 2. All reported adverse events in global safety analysis (%)[18]

	Meloxicam (7.5 mg) (n=893)	Meloxicam (15 mg) (n=3282)	Piroxicam (20 mg) (n=906)	Diclofenac (100 mg) (n=324)	Naproxen (750–1000 mg) (n=243)
Patient-years of exposure	172	1146	166	81	78
Gastrointestinal	17	18	20	27	37
Central nervous system	8	8	7	7	8
Increase in GOT/GPT	6	7	6	16	10
Skin/appendages	7	6	4	4	8
Respiratory system	6	7	4	6	6
Urinary system	4	5	5	3	5
Increase in creatinine/BUN	0.5	0.4	0.9	0.3	0.4
Total	43	45	44	56	61

GOT = glutamate oxalate transaminase; GPT = glutamate pyruvate transaminase; BUN = blood urea nitrogen.

Looking more specifically at the serious GI side effects of perforation, ulceration or bleeding (PUBs) per patient-year of exposure, meloxicam at either dosage appeared safer than the standard NSAIDs (Figure 3). The number of PUBs per 100 patient-years of exposure was numerically lower with meloxicam at either dosage than with piroxicam or naproxen, and meloxicam 7.5 mg was also numerically superior to diclofenac with respect to serious PUBs (i.e. requiring or prolonging hospitalization, or assessed as life-threatening or disabling); no specific statistical analysis was undertaken in this comparison.

Nabumetone 1000 mg daily carries a slightly higher risk of PUB than meloxicam[14,19]; however, this dose is lower than that routinely used in clinical practice

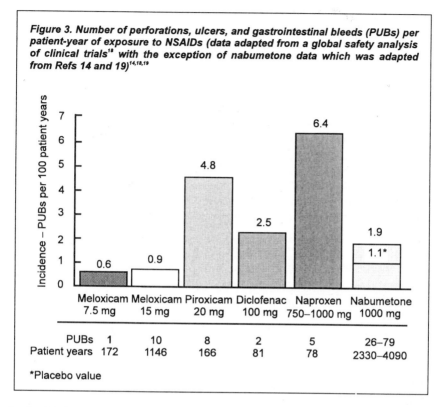

Figure 3. Number of perforations, ulcers, and gastrointestinal bleeds (PUBs) per patient-year of exposure to NSAIDs (data adapted from a global safety analysis of clinical trials[18] with the exception of nabumetone data which was adapted from Refs 14 and 19)[14,18,19]

in the US (1500–2000 mg daily). No safety data are available on the higher doses of nabumetone but raising the dose of an NSAID may be expected to raise the incidence of GI side effects.

Effect on renal function

Many patients who require NSAID treatment are elderly and may have impaired renal function. This can give rise to concerns both about toxicity as a result of reduced excretion of the drug and further impairment of renal function arising as a result of inhibition of physiological renal PG synthesis (a COX-1 mediated function). Meloxicam is almost entirely converted to inactive metabolites prior to excretion and thus is, at least theoretically, well-suited for the elderly[20]. Only very small quantities are excreted unchanged in the urine (<0.25%) and faeces (1.6%)[21].

Reassurance was provided by a 28-day open study of meloxicam 15 mg daily in patients with rheumatic disease and mild renal failure (creatinine clearance 25–60 ml/min)[22]. No significant change in creatinine clearance, serum N-acetyl-β-glucosaminidase/creatinine ratio (a marker of renal tubular damage) or serum urea or potassium occurred over the 28-day duration of the study. Serial measurements of trough levels of meloxicam failed to show any evidence of drug accumulation. In studies of meloxicam in OA (n = 1820) and RA (n = 1889) in patients with normal renal function, the incidence of impaired renal function developing during treatment (creatinine > 1.8 mg/dl or blood urea nitrogen >40 mg/dl) was 0.4%: approximately the same as diclofenac (0.3%) and naproxen (0.4%) but less than piroxicam (0.9%)[18]. RA patients are generally known to experience a higher rate of renal adverse events with NSAIDs than OA patients. When patients with RA were considered separately, piroxicam caused abnormal renal function in 1.6% of patients compared with 0.4% of OA patients; with meloxicam the same incidence (0.4%) was found in both RA and OA groups. In separate studies, etodolac raised creatinine levels in 0.9% of patients whereas nabumetone appeared to have no effect[23,24].

The renal safety profile of meloxicam approximates to that of other NSAIDs in clinical use. It should be possible to use full dosage in patients with mild to moderate renal failure without fear of accumulation or further deterioration in renal function. Patients with end-stage renal failure may have a higher proportion of free (unbound) drug in the plasma, and it may therefore be prudent to use the lower dose of 7.5 mg daily for these patients.

Effect on transaminase levels

Diclofenac 100 mg caused elevation of the serum transaminase levels to over twice the upper limit of normal in approximately 5% of patients in the global analysis of the meloxicam clinical trials programme[18]. This effect was seen in only 2% or less of patients taking naproxen, piroxicam, or either dose of meloxicam.

CONCLUSIONS

A large volume of experimental data is now available to evaluate both the efficacy of meloxicam in RA and OA and its safety profile. When compared with other NSAIDs used in the treatment of OA, meloxicam 7.5 mg daily is as effective as diclofenac 100 mg daily and etodolac 600 mg daily. It is numerically more effective than nabumetone 1000 mg daily, although higher doses of nabumetone are normally used in clinical practice. In RA, the data show that the lower dose of meloxicam of 7.5 mg daily and the higher dose of 15 mg daily are as effective as naproxen 750 mg daily and piroxicam 20 mg daily, respectively.

With regard to the safety of meloxicam, either dose exhibits a GI safety profile which is superior to those of piroxicam 20 mg, naproxen 750–1000 mg, and diclofenac 100 mg for severe side effects such as PUBs, and probably better than that of nabumetone 1000 mg daily. In the renal system, meloxicam is at least as well tolerated as naproxen and diclofenac, and as well tolerated as either piroxicam or etodolac. Nabumetone 1000 mg looks as good, or numerically better than, meloxicam in this system. Diclofenac has a greater propensity to cause elevation of serum transaminases than any other NSAID.

Taken together, these results show that meloxicam has a good safety and efficacy profile, with some indication of increased GI safety over several other NSAIDs. The possible explanation for this profile is meloxicam's relatively selective inhibition of COX-2, enabling it to inhibit potentially pathological prostaglandin synthesis at sites of inflammation but sparing what is thought to be 'physiological' prostaglandin synthesis in the stomach and kidneys.

References

1. Pairet M, Engelhardt G. Distinct isoforms (COX-1 and COX-2) of cyclooxygenase: possible physiological and therapeutic implications. Fundam Clin Pharmacol. 1996; 10: 1–15.
2. Engelhardt G, Bögel R, Schnitzler Chr, Utzmann R. Meloxicam: influence on arachidonic acid metabolism. Biochem Pharmacol. 1996; 51: 21–8.
3. Meade EA, Smith WL, DeWitt DL. Differential inhibition of prostaglandin endoperoxide synthase (cyclooxygenase) isozymes by aspirin and other non-steroidal anti-inflammatory drugs. J Biol Chem. 1993; 268: 6610–14.
4. Churchill L, Graham AG, Shih C-K, Pauletti D, Farina PR, Grob PM. Selective inhibition of human cyclo-oxygenase-2 by meloxicam. Inflammopharmacology. 1996; 4: 125–35.
5. Glaser K, Sung ML, O'Neill K et al. Etodolac selectively inhibits human prostaglandin G/H synthase 2 (PGHS-2) versus human PGHS-1. Eur J Pharmacol. 1995; 281: 107–11.
6. Glaser KB. Cyclooxygenase selectivity and NSAIDs. Cyclooxygenase-2 selectivity of etodolac (Lodine). Inflammopharmacology. 1995; 3: 335–45.
7. Patrignani P, Panara MR, Santini G et al. Differential inhibition of the cyclooxygenase activity of prostaglandin endoperoxide synthase isozymes in vitro and ex vivo in man. Prostaglandins Leukot Essent Fatty Acids. 1996; 55 (Suppl 1): 98.
8. Patrignani P, Panara MR, Greco A et al. Biochemical and pharmacological characterization of the cyclooxygenase activity of human blood prostaglandin endoperoxide synthases. J Pharmacol Exp Ther. 1994; 271: 1705–12.
9. Pairet M, Engelhardt G. Differential inhibition of COX-1 and COX-2 in vitro and pharmacological profile in vivo of NSAIDs. In: Vane J, Botting J, Botting R (eds). Improved Non-steroid Anti-inflammatory Drugs – COX-2 Enzyme Inhibitors. Dordrecht Kluwer Academic Publishers. 1996: 103–19.
10. Stichtenoth DO, Wagner B, Frölich JC. Effects of meloxicam and indomethacin on cyclooxygenase pathways in healthy volunteers. Paper presented at the Biomedicine '96 meeting of the AAP, ASCI, and AFCR in Washington DC, 3–6 May 1996.
11. Hosie J, Distel M, Bluhmki E. Meloxicam in osteoarthritis: a 6-month, double-blind comparison with diclofenac sodium. Br J Rheumatol. 1996; 35 (Suppl 1): 39–43.
12. Platt PN. Recent clinical experience with etodolac in the treatment of osteoarthritis of the knee. Clin Rheumatol. 1989; 8 (Suppl 1): 54–62.
13. Lucker PW, Pawlowski C, Friedrich I, Faiella F, Magni E. Double-blind, randomised, multicentre clinical study evaluating the efficacy and tolerability of nimesulide in comparison with etodolac in patients suffering from osteoarthritis of the knee. Eur J Rheumatol Inflam. 1994; 14: 29–38.
14. Fleischmann RM. Clinical efficacy and safety of nabumetone in rheumatoid arthritis and osteoarthritis. J Rheumatol. 1992; 19 (Suppl 36): 32–40.
15. Wojtulewski JA, Schattenkirchner M, Barceló P et al. A six-month double-blind trial to compare the efficacy and safety of meloxicam 7.5 mg daily and naproxen 750 mg daily in patients with rheumatoid arthritis. Br J Rheumatol. 1996; 35 (Suppl 1): 22–8.
16. Huskisson EC, Narjes H, Bluhmki E, Degner F. Comparison of meloxicam 15 mg and piroxicam 20 mg in a 3-week, double-blind trial in RA. Eighth APLAR Congress of Rheumatology, Melbourne, 1996. Abstract no. 351.
17. Patoia L. Santucci L, Furno P et al. A 4-week, double-blind, parallel-group study to compare the gastrointestinal effects of meloxicam 7.5 mg, meloxicam 15 mg, piroxicam 20 mg and placebo by means of faecal blood loss, endoscopy and symptom evaluation in healthy volunteers. Br J Rheumatol. 1996; 35 (Suppl 1): 61–7.
18. Distel M, Mueller C, Bluhmki E, Fries J. Safety of meloxicam: A global analysis of clinical trials. Br J Rheumatol. 1996; 35 (Suppl 1): 68–77.
19. Jackson RE, Mitchell FN, Brindley DA. Safety evaluation of nabumetone in United States clinical trials. Am J Med. 1987; 83: 115–20.

20. Schmid J, Busch U, Trummlitz G, Prox A, Kaschke S, Wachsmuth H. Meloxicam: Metabolic profile and biotransformation products in the rat. Xenobiotica. 1995; 25: 1219–36.
21. Türck D, Roth W, Busch U. A review of the clinical pharmacokinetics of meloxicam. Br J Rheumatol. 1996; 35 (Suppl 1): 13–16.
22. Bevis PFR, Bird HA, Lapham G. An open study to assess the safety and tolerability of meloxicam 15 mg in subjects with rheumatic disease and mild renal impairment. Br J Rheumatol. 1996; 35 (Suppl 1): 56–60.
23. Shand DG, Epstein C, Kinberg-Calhoun J, Mullane JF, Sanda M. The effect of etodolac administration on renal function in patients with arthritis. J Clin Pharmacol. 1986; 26: 269–74.
24. Aronoff GR. Therapeutic implications associated with renal studies of nabumetone. J Rheumatol. 1992; 19 (Suppl 36): 25–31.

Index

A549 cells 57, 61–2
adrenic acid 60
Alzheimer's disease 5, 47, 52
amino acid residues 24
γ-aminobutyric acid 49
analgesic nephropathy 87
angioedema, isolated periorbital 104
angiotensin-II 88, 122
antidiuretic hormone (vasopressin) 88, 89, 90–1
anti-sense oligonucleotides 56
APC gene 4
apoptosis 55–64
  cyclooxygenases and 55
arachidonate 74
arachidonic acid 1, 2, 50, 60
  free 48
  substrate 127
aryl methyl sulphonamide compounds 24
ascites 88
aspirin 1, 2, 5, 61
  adverse reactions 100–1
  antithrombotic effects 74
  colon cancer effect 3–4
  COX inhibitor 56
  gastrointestinal toxicity 73
  high dose 57
  low dose 73–4
aspirin-induced asthma 99–104
  corticoids role 101
  COX theory 100–1
  early studies 100
  leukotriene hypothesis 103–4
  PGD_2 hypothesis 102–3
  PGE_2 hypothesis 101–2
  $PGF_{2\alpha}$ hypothesis 102–3
  viral hypothesis 102
aspirin-like drugs 2
  new classification 109–15
asthma 5–6, 99–104
  aspirin-induced see aspirin-induced asthma
  aspirin-relieved 104

aspirin-tolerant 99
autoimmune vasculitis 104

Baltimore Longitudinal Study of Ageing 5
Bartter's syndrome 88
B cell apoptosis 55
benign neoplasm apoptosis 59
benzfurans 119
bioactive lipids 48–50
BN 52021 49
BN 50730 50, 51
bovine aortic endothelial cells 29
brain 3, 4

carageenin pleurisy 93
catecholamines 88
β-catenin 59
celecoxib (SC-58635) 8, 9–10, 74, 94, 119
  efficacy in man 130–1
  structure 10 (fig.)
cell cycle regulators 59–60
cell-free systems 110
cerebral cortex 4
cerebral ischaemia 48, 52
cerebrovascular diseases 52
choronic gonadotrophin 6
Churg–Strauss syndrome (granulomatous angiitis) 104
cigarette smoking 74
CI-1004 11–12
c-myc expression 56
colorectal cancer 67, 70
  aspirin effect 3, 67
  cell lines 61
  COX-2 activity 70
  deaths in USA 71
  familial syndromes 71
compound (7) (DFU) 119
corticosteroids 2
COX 1
  active site 1–2
  apoptosis regulation 56